The Black Woman's Breast Cancer Survival Guide

The Black Woman's Breast Cancer Survival Guide

Understanding and Healing in the Face of a Nationwide Crisis

Cheryl D. Holloway

Foreword by Philip Agop Philip, MD, PhD, FRCP

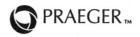

PRAEGER™

An Imprint of ABC-CLIO, LLC

Santa Barbara, California • Denver, Colorado

This book discusses treatments (including types of medication and mental health therapies), diagnostic tests for various symptoms and mental health disorders, and organizations. The author has made every effort to present accurate and up-to-date information. However, the information in this book is not intended to recommend or endorse particular treatments or organizations, or substitute for the care or medical advice of a qualified health professional, or used to alter any medical therapy without a medical doctor's advice. Specific situations may require specific therapeutic approaches not included in this book. For those reasons, we recommend that readers follow the advice of qualified healthcare professionals directly involved in their care. Readers who suspect they may have specific medical problems should consult a physician about any suggestions made in this book.

Library of Congress Cataloging-in-Publication Data

Names: Holloway, Cheryl D., author.
Title: The black woman's breast cancer survival guide : understanding and
    healing in the face of a nationwide crisis / Cheryl D. Holloway ; foreword
    by Philip Agop Philip, MD.
Description: Santa Barbara, California : Praeger, an imprint of ABC-CLIO,
    LLC, [2017] | Includes bibliographical references and index.
Identifiers: LCCN 2017009519 (print) | LCCN 2017010693 (ebook) |
    ISBN 9781440856082 (alk.paper) | ISBN 9781440856099 (eISBN)
Subjects: LCSH: Breast—Cancer. | African American women—Health and hygiene. |
    Breast—Cancer—Treatment. | African American women—Medical care.
Classification: LCC RC280.B8 H635 2017 (print) | LCC RC280.B8 (ebook) |
    DDC 616.99/449—dc23
LC record available at https://lccn.loc.gov/2017009519

ISBN: 978-1-4408-5608-2
EISBN: 978-1-4408-5609-9

21 20 19 18 17   2 3 4 5

This book is also available as an eBook.

Praeger
An Imprint of ABC-CLIO, LLC

ABC-CLIO, LLC
130 Cremona Drive, P.O. Box 1911
Santa Barbara, California 93116-1911
www.abc-clio.com

This book is printed on acid-free paper ∞

Manufactured in the United States of America

Contents

Foreword   vii
　　by Philip Agop Philip, MD, PhD, FRCP

Acknowledgments   ix

Introduction   xi

Part One　　**Dealing with the Basics for Black Women**   1

Chapter 1　Why Black Women Need to Pay Close
　　　　　　Attention to Cancer and Cancer Screening   3

Chapter 2　Dealing with Common Emotions and
　　　　　　Talking to Others   30

Chapter 3　Types of Breast Cancer Black Women May Develop   49

Part Two　　**Understanding Cancer Test Results**   65

Chapter 4　Breast Cancer Health Screens   67

Chapter 5　Understanding Cancer Test Results   79

Part Three　**What You Need to Know about Breast
　　　　　　　Cancer Treatment**   93

Chapter 6　Surgery   95

Chapter 7　Radiation Therapy   114

Chapter 8　Chemotherapy, Anti-Estrogen (Endocrine) Therapy,
　　　　　　Combined Therapies, and Emerging Treatments   128

Chapter 9   Watching Out for Other Forms of Cancer   146

Chapter 10   Cancer Is Gone: Be Happy—But Don't Let
                  Your Guard Down   160

Conclusion   171

Appendix A: Organizations That Can Help   175

Appendix B: Other Websites with Helpful Information   177

Appendix C: Glossary   179

Bibliography   187

Index   195

Foreword

Philip Agop Philip, MD, PhD, FRCP

I'm an oncologist in Detroit who has treated hundreds of women with breast cancer and I would be ecstatic if a cure for this disease were discovered very soon, preferably today or next week. Undoubtedly the cure rates for women who have breast cancer diagnosed in its earlier stages are increasing provided they are diagnosed early and are provided the right treatment. However, a significant proportion of patients are still diagnosed in more advanced stages or their cancer returns after an initial diagnosis of early-stage breast cancer. Those women with advanced breast cancer are rarely cured with current available therapies. A cure for breast cancer would benefit women of all races, but especially would be a boon for black women, who are more prone to developing aggressive tumors that can be very challenging for physicians like me to treat successfully. This is why I strongly recommend Dr. Holloway's book that you are about to read. Let me be very clear. If you are a black woman with breast cancer, you need the information in this book whether you are diagnosed with an early-stage or a more advanced breast cancer. In addition, if you are a person interested in the problems faced by black women with breast cancer, you also need to read this book. No other book concentrates exclusively on black women and their breast cancer issues. Dr. Holloway is herself a black woman who has faced breast cancer twice, and she knows how it feels from the inside out. She is also an excellent researcher. Consequently, this book provides both practical and invaluable heartfelt advice.

The Black Woman's Breast Cancer Survival Guide: Understanding and Healing in the Face of a Nationwide Crisis is a uniquely valuable book because it summarizes and explains the findings of clear-eyed research demonstrating that, far too often, black women have significantly worse prognoses with their diagnosis, treatment, and outcomes of breast cancer than white women, a finding that distresses Dr. Holloway and worries me as well. I hope that physicians and other healthcare professionals also read this book because I think there is a lack of awareness about the challenges black women with breast cancer face. I also hope that this book may convince researchers to perform more studies on the existing racial disparities in breast cancer. Because only then we can work on zeroing in on the underlying causes for these differences and create the right solutions for black women who face breast cancer in the future—among them, your daughters, your mother, your sisters, your cousins, your nieces, your friends, and other women.

This book fulfills several key missions. It offers the most recent information on the diagnosis of and treatments for women with breast cancer, with particular concern for the issues affecting black women. The book also provides the important questions all women with breast cancer should ask their physicians, and urges them to *not* be shrinking violets when it comes to asking questions about their bodies in general and regarding their breast cancer in particular. Too many women are far too intimidated by their physicians and they fail to ask questions when they don't understand something and are confused. Please, ask those questions! Oncologists, at least *this* oncologist, want you to know everything you need to know to improve your odds for recovery.

I would also like to add that I think too many patients go to their oncology appointments alone, without a friend or a family member to stand by them and provide another pair of listening ears. Cancer is a devastating diagnosis and it's hard to be a good listener when you are hearing about surgery, radiation, or chemotherapy, as well as what stage the cancer is and so forth. Bring a pad of paper or even a voice recorder with you and ask your family member or friend to bring one too. Take notes and ask your doctor all the questions that you can think of.

This comprehensive book also discusses what to say about your breast cancer to others, and how to respond to the often-intrusive questions many people ask you, such as if cancer could be God's punishment for something you did or failed to do in the past. I agree with Dr. Holloway when she says that God made oncologists to treat people with cancer. The book also talks about dealing with side effects from surgery, chemotherapy, radiation treatments, or other therapies. Once you finish this book, you will have a good basic understanding of breast cancer and you may wish to return to some chapters again as you have different treatments or encounter some of the side effects of treatment.

I wholeheartedly recommend Dr. Holloway's book and I wish good health to all readers. Let us all continue to fervently hope for a cure for breast cancer.

Acknowledgments

I dedicate this book to the memory of my mother, Alberta, whose hard work and determination encouraged me to become the woman I am today. She taught me to strive to reach greater heights in life, to remember the roads that I have traveled and the bridges I have crossed, and to reach out, touch, and help someone along the way.

Special thanks to Dr. Philip Agop Philip, who was my guide through breast cancer when I did not know which direction to go and how this disease would impact my life. I am forever grateful to God for placing Dr. Philip in my life as my oncologist and assisting me with this survival guide for all black women to have the knowledge and understanding about breast cancer, treatment, and life with and after breast cancer.

Thank you to Dr. Donald Weaver, who has been with me from the very start of my journey with breast cancer. It was Dr. Weaver who advised me, when I was first diagnosed, to do all that I can medically and to let God do the rest. I believe it was God who placed Dr. Weaver in my life to perform the many successful surgeries I have had over the years, and for that I am truly grateful.

Thank you to Dr. Washington, who was my amazing radiation oncologist. It was Dr. Washington who educated me on the process and importance of chemotherapy. She encouraged me while addressing many of my fears and concerns about how this therapy would impact one's body. As a result of her compassion and extensive knowledge, I ended up choosing life over losing my hair, which grew back even healthier than before.

Finally, thanks to my daughter Erika and my son Clay for all of their love, assistance, and encouragement to share my knowledge of breast cancer and experiences with other women.

Introduction

A breast cancer diagnosis is a terrifying experience, and a woman who hears that she has breast cancer needs all the help she can get. This is especially true for black women, who are more likely than all other races and ethnicities to develop a fast-growing type of breast cancer when they are in their childbearing years. I am a black woman and also a three-time cancer survivor who has learned valuable lessons that I will share with you in this book. I am also adept at academic research, and have scoured research databases for studies that would be particularly useful to you in your own quest to overcome breast cancer. My goal is to provide you with the information that you need to deal with your breast cancer, as well as to cope with all the emotions that surround it.

I have survived two bouts with breast cancer and have also survived thyroid cancer that was probably caused by my radiation treatments for breast cancer. I am also living proof that when cancer is identified, death does not have to be immediate or inevitable. Of course, death itself *is* ultimately inevitable for us all, but this does *not* mean that a cancer diagnosis leads in a direct path to dying young. Sadly, however, far too many young and middle-aged black women die from breast cancer, and that is why I wrote this book. They die unnecessarily because their cancer is not diagnosed in time or because they refuse to seek treatment that is readily available in the form of surgery, radiation, chemotherapy, and other options. They die because of lack of access to health care or lack of knowledge of available resources that many minorities are not aware are available to assist them in their diagnosis and treatment of cancer. They die because they did not know that they had a family history of breast cancer, because no one wanted to talk about that mother, grandmother, aunt, uncle, brother, sister, and cousin who died of cancer—or maybe nobody in the family knew that family members died from breast cancer because they never went to the doctor to even know they had cancer. They die because they may see a cancer diagnosis as a punishment for real or imagined sins, and they believe they must docilely accept this fate. I don't agree with that choice and that is why I wrote this book for black women.

Cancer is the adversary. When you receive a cancer diagnosis, remember that it is not your body that is turning against you. Instead, it is cancer itself that is trying to destroy your body, and I strongly believe that you need to fight back. As a Christian woman, I believe that God has placed cancer doctors (oncologists) on this earth to help people be treated for breast cancer and other types of cancer. There are many types of treatments that are options, and each woman needs a specific treatment tailored to eradicate the type of cancer in her body. That is why you need to listen to your oncologist and carefully consider what he or she is saying. If you don't like the doctor, get a second opinion. But don't use not liking your doctor as an excuse to delay receiving treatment to fight your cancer adversary.

Another problem lies within part of the establishment itself. Black women are more likely to get cancer in their childbearing years than women of other races and ethnicities, and even to get breast cancer when they are younger than the age of 40. Yet major organizations such as the American Cancer Society say that women, all women, don't need mammograms until after age 45. Other medical experts recommend mammogram screening start at age 40. But if I had waited to receive my first mammogram when I was 45 years old or even 40, I would not have lived long enough to experience that mammogram, because my breast cancer was diagnosed when I was just 38. It was severe enough that I needed surgery, radiation, and chemotherapy to get rid of the cancer. That was about 20 years ago, and I'm still here, and still spreading the word about breast cancer in churches and other locations.

I think the medical establishment should encourage black women to receive their first baseline mammogram when they are 35 years old or younger, especially if there is a known family history of breast cancer. (And if you don't know if anyone in your family has ever had breast cancer, ask them! Tell them you need this information to protect yourself and your other female relatives, and it's not something you want to gossip about to others.)

White women are diagnosed more with breast cancer than black women, but black women tend to develop more aggressive tumors than white women and at an earlier age, which results in both more severe sickness and higher death rates. So, I think that the new guideline recommendations to hold off on mammograms until they are 45 should be changed for black women.

African American women need to stand up and, if necessary, insist on getting mammograms starting when they are in their thirties. Sure, nobody likes mammograms. Experts say that they are "discomforting," but let's face it, they actually do hurt. But dying young because of breast cancer and leaving your children without a mother and dying before you can fulfill your purpose in life is a much worse fate than a few minutes of pain from a mammogram.

In this book, I talk about some of the possible reasons why black women are more prone to develop dangerous and life-threatening forms of breast cancer than white women or women of other races and ethnicities. I also talk about the importance of telling others who are key people in your life that you have breast cancer, and how to deal with some of the completely unreasonable things that some people will say to you, such as, "Have you sinned?" I am not joking about this: I was personally told that I had developed cancer because I was not close enough to God. I believe in God, but I don't think that God gives women breast cancer to punish them.

The book also covers what breast cancer is, how it is diagnosed, and how it's treated, whether by surgery, radiation, chemotherapy or a combination of therapies or other treatments. I also discuss some other forms of cancer that are common among black women, such as lung cancer. I sincerely hope that you will find my book interesting and helpful, and that it provides you with the information that you need. At a minimum, I hope that my book educates you and energizes you to obtain the treatment that you need. Do not give up and do not be passive in your struggle. This is a battle and you *must* go into *survival mode*. Whenever you can, do what is needed to save your life from the cancer enemy. Don't let it win. Fight back.

Cheryl Holloway, PhD

PART 1

Dealing with the Basics for Black Women

Part One is made up of three separate chapters covering some of the basics you need to know about breast cancer. In Chapter One, I explain why black women especially need to know about and pay attention to breast cancer. Chapter Two covers the common emotions that women feel when they receive a breast cancer diagnosis and discusses talking to your significant other (husband, boyfriend, girlfriend, wife) about your cancer diagnosis, which is a very difficult and painful step for many women. It is so painful that some of them forego telling others at all, robbing themselves of the comfort and care of the people who love them. Chapter Three describes the different types of breast cancer, which is important information you need to know.

CHAPTER ONE

Why Black Women Need to Pay Close Attention to Cancer and Cancer Screening

Hearing that you have breast cancer is a uniquely frightening experience that often feels like time has suddenly stopped because you are engulfed within a paralyzing terror. It's sort of like being frozen in time, and it's hard to listen to anyone or even think a coherent thought because someone has just told you that you have the "C word"—cancer. In the real world, however, time keeps ticking away despite how you feel, and despite your shock, fear, panic, and all the many other emotions that you may experience when you hear about your extremely distressing life-changing diagnosis.

You might be really scared even before you hear the diagnosis. When my mammogram was finished and the doctor came in to say that he needed "a few more pictures," my heart sunk. I feared that it was cancer, and I was right. I have had breast cancer twice in my life, and each time that I heard the diagnosis, it felt like being kicked in the stomach or maybe in the head. But I'm a fighter, and I worked with my doctor on the treatment plan each time and followed it through all the way. After I recovered from each incident of breast cancer, I decided that I needed to share information about breast cancer with other women, which is why I became a volunteer for the American Cancer Society. It is also why I did my doctoral dissertation on the attitudes and behavior toward screening for breast cancer among young black women. In addition, my desire to share information with others is also why I wrote this book.

Cancer is a tough disease. The treatments themselves can be very debilitating. You may feel like you're David facing the Goliath of cancer, except you don't have a slingshot to bring you certain victory. I can't take away all your fear. But I can give you a lot of information and help within these pages, and I can also offer you other resources where you can find more assistance to cope with your breast cancer.

Why Black Women Need Their Own Breast Cancer Book

You may wonder why black women need their own book on breast cancer. If I wanted to write a book about breast cancer, why didn't I just write about breast cancer for all women? After all, cancer is cancer and *it* doesn't know if you're black, white, Hispanic, a Pacific Islander, or any other race or ethnicity, right? Maybe. But then again, maybe not. Here's why.

A lot of people don't realize that black women are more likely than women of all other races or ethnicities to be diagnosed with dangerous and rapidly spreading forms of breast cancer, such as triple-negative breast cancer or inflammatory breast cancer.[1] In addition, black women are more likely to develop breast cancer before age 40 than any other group.[2] And last, and probably most frightening, black women with breast cancer are the most likely to die from breast cancer, based on multiple large-scale studies.[3] Making it even worse, black women who are young (under age 40 or 50, depending on the study) are more likely to die from breast cancer than women of other races and ethnicities who are diagnosed with breast cancer when they are young.[4] For example, in a large-scale study of nearly 163,000 women under age 50 who were diagnosed with breast cancer, which included about 127,000 whites, 20,000 blacks and 16,000 people of other races, researcher Foluso O. Ademuywa and colleagues found that the five-year survival rate from breast cancer was 90 percent for whites and 79 percent for blacks.[5] The five-year survival rate refers to women who were alive five years after they were first diagnosed with breast cancer. This is a significant and scary 11-point difference, and yet another reason why black women need their own book on breast cancer.

As a breast cancer survivor myself as well as a college professor, I became curious about the reasons *why* black women with breast cancer are faring so poorly compared to women of other races, and so I started amassing the research information that I report and explain to you in this book. I also read all the other books on breast cancer, and either they never mentioned black women at all or they dedicated maybe a paragraph on the subject. That isn't good enough! I am black myself and

I was shocked to learn the facts I've already stated. Sometimes when nothing is out there that helps a group that really matters to you, like black women with breast cancer matter to me, then you have to stand up and do the job yourself. That's why I wrote this book for black women with breast cancer.

In the recent past, there were fewer cases of black women with breast cancer than white women, although they had higher death rates. But research published in 2016 by Carol E. DeSantis and her colleagues[6] and

---

BLACK WOMEN AND GENETICS

In 2016, the National Institutes of Health announced that it had launched the largest study ever on breast cancer genetics among black women. The Breast Cancer Genetic Study in African-Ancestry Populations Initiative will compare the genetic makeup of 20,000 black women with breast cancer to the genetics of 20,000 black women who do not have breast cancer, looking for disparities and similarities. The study will also compare the genetics of black women with breast cancer to the genetics of white women who also have breast cancer.

It is hoped that this study will provide important information that can help decrease the high death rate among black women with breast cancer.

It's about time that such a study was made, because researchers have used genetic material from black people for years, sometimes (probably often!) without permission. Did you know that the HeLa cells, which have been the basis for genetic research for more than 50 years, were originally taken from the cancerous cervical tumor of a poor black woman at Johns Hopkins Hospital in Baltimore, Maryland, back in 1951? Her name was Henrietta Lacks, and the researchers who excised her tissue began growing her cells for experimentation, unbeknownst to her, and these cells still live on in the 21st century. Henrietta Lacks's cells have shown amazing longevity and they have lived longer than Ms. Lacks herself, who died of cancer in 1951. Her unique cells were used to develop genetic mapping and have also been used in cancer research as well as research in many other medical fields. For example, they were used to develop the polio vaccine. Lacks's story is described in the best-selling book by Rebecca Skloot, *The Immortal Life of Henrietta Lacks.*[1]

[1]Rebecca Skloot, *The Immortal Life of Henrietta Lacks* (New York: Crown Publishers, 2010).

also by Anne Marie McCarthy[7] revealed that, starting in 2012, the breast cancer rate among black women was converging to about the same rate as found among white women. Even more shockingly, the researchers found that black women are 42 percent more likely to die of breast cancer than were white women.[8] This is likely due to fast-developing cancers as well as to diagnoses at more advanced stages of cancer. Genetic predispositions also likely play a major role.

I've offered some rather gloomy statistics in Chapter One, but these negative numbers don't mean that if you have breast cancer and you are also black, then you should abandon all hope. Not at all! My book is meant as a message of hope for you. This book offers you practical and useful information as well as hopeful information too.

Mammograms: Black Women Need Them at Younger Ages

Here's another problem and yet another reason why black women need their own book on breast cancer, which I alluded to in my Introduction. In case you missed this point, I need to tell you again that most doctors and insurance companies advise against mammogram screenings for women under age 40, no matter what their race is. But what about black women who develop breast cancer when they are younger than age 40? I was 38 years old when my breast cancer was diagnosed. I specifically requested a mammogram, and my doctor agreed to write a prescription for the procedure. If I had waited, I could have died before I ever reached age 40. This is important not just to me but also to other black women, who are more likely to develop breast cancer at younger ages than women of all other races and ethnicities.

I want to sound a clarion call not only to women who know that they have breast cancer but also to women who *may* have breast cancer that screening with a mammogram would reveal. And I also want to encourage black women who are diagnosed with breast cancer to tell others about it. Yet the tide is turning toward later and later screening for breast cancer, which may be very ominous for black women.

What's the scope of the problem? According to the American Cancer Society, nearly 31,000 black women will develop breast cancer in 2016, so we can assume at least this number will develop breast cancer in subsequent years—if not more. Breast cancer is the most common type of cancer that black women develop.[9] Obviously, not every black woman will develop breast cancer. There are health risk factors for this disease and I will explain to you what they are in this chapter. There are also behavioral risk factors as well, which also I discuss in this chapter. Keep in mind, however, that you may not fit into these risk categories that I describe and yet you could still be diagnosed with breast cancer. I know you don't want to hear that, but sadly, it's the truth. Forewarned is forearmed. Get that annual mammogram.

Breast Cancer Is a Disease, Not an Embarrassment

If you have breast cancer, I highly recommend that you tell your family members, your friends, and the people whom you work with. If you do so, then you are likely to save at least five lives by spreading the word about breast cancer and the benefit of mammograms. I know that I have saved lives, because when I spoke out about the need to have a mammogram in churches and at other places, women called me later to say that they were glad they had the mammogram, because they were diagnosed with breast cancer and now they could be treated. I suspect that black women may be much more reticent about telling others about their breast cancer diagnosis than white women, probably for many reasons, and two of those reasons are guilt and shame. But my attitude is this: We need to talk about it. The more knowledge and awareness we all have, the better future we can expect. So, if you have breast cancer, then ask your mother if she had breast cancer and ask your sisters, your cousins, your aunts, and your grandma. You might think they would have mentioned this fact to you, and you could be wrong. But breast cancer is nobody's fault.

Also, whenever possible, please get genetic testing. It appears to me that research is converging on a likely genetic cause of breast cancer. So, although I talk about factors like obesity and smoking that can increase your risk for breast cancer, your genetic makeup is extremely important too. In fact, it may be the key reason why black women have such high rates of breast cancer compared to women of other races. For example, some studies have found the same kind of breast cancer in African women (in countries in the continent of Africa) as they have found in black women of similar ancestry in the United States, a fact I'll discuss later in this book.[10] Knowing about your genes is also important because the type of treatment that you need is often directly linked to the genetics of your tumor. Yet many black women don't have genetic testing, which is a major mistake that needs to be rectified. At a minimum, the breast tumor should be genetically tested to help determine the best treatment.

BLACK FEMALE BREAST CANCER DEATH RATE
IS MUCH HIGHER IN SOME CITIES

It's bad enough that black women have a higher death rate from breast cancer than women of other races and ethnicities. But the death risks from this form of cancer are even higher in some cities, based on recent research findings.

A study reported in the Journal *Cancer Epidemiology* in 2014 by Bijou R. Hunt and colleagues found that death ratios among black women with breast cancer were significantly higher in some cities for the period 2005–2009.[1] To understand this statistic simply, if black women died at the same ratio as white women, the ratio would be 1.00 or 1 to 1. If black women died at a higher rate, the number would be greater than 1.00, and if they died at a lower rate, then the ratio would be less than 1.00.

For example, in considering the 50 largest cities in the United States, the researchers found that in Memphis, Tennessee (the worst city for black female breast cancer deaths, with a ratio of 2.11), black women with breast cancer were more than twice as likely to die from breast cancer as were white women with breast cancer. The next highest breast cancer death rates among black women were found in Los Angeles, California, where the ratio was 1.71 and Wichita, Kansas, where the ratio was 1.57. The national rate for black women dying from breast cancer was 1.4.

Interestingly, in some cities, the death rate from breast cancer for black and white women was about the *same,* as in Las Vegas, Nevada, Virginia Beach, Virginia, and Sacramento, California. No one knows exactly why black women are dying from breast cancer at a higher rate in some cities than others or why the rate is about the same as white women in other cities, but it certainly seems like a subject worthy of more research. Possibly the issue is related to socioeconomic status and/or healthcare access.

[1] Bijou Hunt, Steve Whitman, and Marc S. Hurlbert, "Increasing Black: White Disparities in Breast Cancer Mortality in the 50 Largest Cities in the United States," *Cancer Epidemiology* 38 (2014): 118–123.

Treatment of Black Women

Okay, maybe I have convinced you now that black women should be concerned about breast cancer and should be sure to get an annual mammogram. But perhaps I have not yet convinced you that black women need a book that includes information on treatment for breast cancer. I have a case for this issue as well.

Some research shows that black women do not fare as well in their hospital treatment for breast cancer than do white women or women of other races, although the reasons why this is true are unclear.[11] It could be that the black breast cancer patients are sicker than the patients of other races or ethnicities. Or it could be that there are still some rudiments of racism left in our society that need to be weeded out. Just because we had a black president of the United States for eight years doesn't mean that racism is dead and gone forever. However, it's also true that sometimes race *does* need to be taken into consideration, especially when it comes to health issues such as breast cancer, which is not an equal opportunity disease. What I mean is that breast cancer does not strike women of all races and ethnicities in the same way. In many cases, breast cancer is worse for black women, which means earlier diagnosis and treatment is crucial. Yet groups like the American Cancer Society, an organization that I love and have done volunteer work with for years, say that all women ages 45–54 years should start getting mammograms every year, while women ages 40–44 may have annual mammograms if they wish to do so. Even worse, the U.S. Preventive Task Force, a group of medical professionals that creates national screening guidelines, recommends starting mammograms at age 50![12] These ages of 45 or 50 years for starting mammograms do not take into account that black women who get breast cancer often develop aggressive tumors at a younger age than women of other races and ethnicities. Saying that women of all races should start screening mammograms at age 45 years, or worse, age 50, is like saying that black, white, and Asian women all should be screened for sickle cell disease at the same rate. When race is a major factor in a health problem, I strongly believe that it should be taken into consideration.

In my own case, I was first diagnosed with breast cancer at age 38— with a mammogram. The point here is that when a screening test like a mammogram is perceived as "optional," and since most women don't like to get mammograms in the first place, they or their physicians may delay this important screening test until age 45. This also means that a case of breast cancer that could have been diagnosed earlier in a black woman will be missed altogether because of this delay. For this reason, I think all black women should be given an earlier age for recommended (not optional!) mammograms, starting at age 35 or 40, latest.[13] I'd also like to add that the American College of Obstetricians and Gynecologists continues to recommend annual screening with mammograms, starting at age 40.[14] If your primary care doctor won't order a mammogram starting at age 40, ask your gynecologist to order one.

What Is Breast Cancer?

Breast cancer is a malignant tumor that originally starts in the breast, and, if left unidentified and untreated, it will eventually spread to the rest of the body. Breast cancer comprises abnormal cells that rapidly multiply—although the speed of the tumor's growth varies greatly from woman to woman. Healthy cells in your body are constantly being created and dying out, and that's a normal process under tight control. Abnormal cells also develop sometimes but they are usually eliminated by your body's efficient immune system, and you never know that they existed. However, the uncontrolled growth of abnormal cells into a cancerous tumor is very harmful to your body and is likely to kill you if it is not diagnosed and treated. The good news is that treatment is available in the form of surgery, radiation therapy, and chemotherapy. In addition, emerging treatments are also being developed by researchers, such as therapies that will help target and eradicate different types of cancer cells based on their molecular makeup. It is well-recognized that cancer cells have different genetic profiles in different patients and even within the tumor of a patient. This requires tailoring therapies by using the right drug for each patient, which will be a major advance toward personalized medicine. This will not only make treatments much more efficacious but also spare some patients futile therapies. Drugs that minimize the effects of estrogen, the female sex organ, are another option for some forms of breast cancer (hormone receptor positive), although not for triple-negative cancer, a form of breast cancer that is more common in black women.[15]

But before we get to discussing the treatment of breast cancer, you will need to learn about the different types of breast cancer that have been identified today, as well as the types that are more commonly found in black women. There are two common types of breast cancer that may be present in all women, including ductal carcinoma and lobular carcinoma. Some women have a combination of ductal and lobular carcinoma. Rarer forms of cancer, which also appear more commonly in black women, are inflammatory breast cancer and triple-negative breast cancer. Read more about the different types of breast cancer in Chapter Three.

**What *Not* to Do When You Are Diagnosed
with Breast Cancer**

1. Do not let your husband or significant other decide what treatment you should have or not have. Instead, consult with your doctor, learn what you can about cancer, and decide for yourself.

2. Do not listen to people who say it's your fault you got cancer. They may be trying to make you feel bad and certainly they are not helping you at all. Treatment is what you need, not self-recrimination.

3. Do not keep the diagnosis to yourself because you are ashamed or embarrassed about your cancer. This is the time when you need to ask for help from others.

4. Do not decide to wait a few months to think about what to do. After a cancer diagnosis, see an oncologist as soon as possible to learn about your particular cancer problem and possible options you need to consider.

5. Do not listen to your herbalist or psychic (or anyone else) instead of your doctor. Your physician is the expert. If you are wary of your doctor, get a second opinion.

Risk Factors for Breast Cancer

Some black women have a greater risk of developing breast cancer than others. This does not mean that it's their fault that they got cancer. It is merely an explanation that some factors apparently increase the risk for breast cancer (as well as other forms of cancer, such as colorectal cancer or lung cancer). There is nothing that you can do about your genetic makeup. However, if your mother, sister, or aunt had breast cancer, you should definitely be vigilant about seeking a mammogram for yourself.

When you see your primary care doctor or your gynecologist, be sure to tell your doctor about the family health risks that you face, and also report the age of your relative(s) when *diagnosed*. Don't wait for the doctor to ask you. Volunteer the information upfront and make sure she is listening. You can tell if the doctor is listening to you by her response to this information. Doctors usually pay attention when someone tells them that their mother or aunt had breast cancer, especially when that individual was under 50 years of age at the time of the diagnosis.

Sometimes you may need to strongly request that your doctor order a mammogram if you are younger than age 45, based on previously mentioned current standards of ordering mammograms starting at age 45. Not all doctors are aware of the risks that black women face for developing an aggressive form of breast cancer at a younger age than white women. If your primary care doctor won't order a mammogram, then ask your gynecologist to order one. Be sure to tell him too about your family health risks for breast cancer, no matter what your age is. This is valuable information to a physician. In case the doctor does not respond when you report this information, say it again. Also, if you are 38 or 39 and you have a family history of breast cancer—or even if you're just worried that you may have breast cancer—tell your gynecologist, who is the most likely physician to be willing to order a mammogram for you, especially since gynecologists believe all women should start getting mammograms at age 40.

Genetic testing may also be available if there is a family history of breast cancer. *BRCA1* and *BRCA2* testing will determine inherited genetic mutations that may increase your breast cancer risks. These specific genetic mutations refer to Breast Cancer 1 and Breast Cancer 2 mutations. Mutations in the *BRCA1* and *BRCA2* genes are the most common inherited causes of breast cancer. Other rare mutations may also make some women more susceptible to developing breast cancer. Genetic testing reveals the presence of potential genetic problems, particularly in families that have a history of breast cancer. Genetic testing is expensive, however, so often it isn't performed.

Some researchers have looked at genetic issues among black women diagnosed with breast cancer. For example, geneticist Tuya Pal and colleagues at the Moffitt Cancer Center in Tampa, Florida, performed a study of nearly 400 black women from Florida who were known breast cancer survivors. The women were aged 50 years and younger, with an average age of 42 years, and all were drawn from the Florida Cancer Registry. The researchers evaluated these women's DNA, based on their collected saliva samples. The results of this study were published in 2015.[16]

The researchers found that 12 percent (49 women) of the group tested positive for either *BRCA1* or *BRCA2*. The researchers also found that among the women who were diagnosed with breast cancer at age 35 years or younger, 22 percent had either a *BRCA1* or a *BRCA2* mutation. In contrast, only 8 percent of the women of ages 46–50 had these mutations. Clearly, the mutation appears to be more strongly associated with younger black women.

The higher rate that Dr. Pal found of these genetic mutations among black women may be another clue explaining why black women are more likely to develop rapidly growing and dangerous forms of breast cancer.

As a result of their findings, the researchers recommended that all black women diagnosed with breast cancer who are aged 50 years and younger should be tested for these genetic mutations.[17] Yet research has shown that only about half of all black women with breast cancer receive such genetic testing and counseling. Clearly, that percentage needs to increase, particularly among younger black women at high risk for rapidly growing forms of breast cancer. Some key contributing factors may be a lack of public awareness and education, as well as cultural issues and the cost of testing, and people simply not wanting to know that they have cancer.

General Risk Factors for Breast Cancer

Here are some general risk factors for breast cancer among all women, with further information about black women. As mentioned earlier, it's important to keep in mind that, even if you have NONE of the risk factors that are described in this chapter, you can still develop breast cancer. So you could be a skinny nondrinking woman who doesn't smoke, didn't receive high dosages of radiation in the past, and have no relatives who ever had breast cancer—as far as you know. This is another reason why all women should be screened for breast cancer. The known risk factors for breast cancer are as follows:

- Obesity
- Genetics: female family members who had breast cancer or a related cancer, such as ovarian cancer, or a male family member who has had breast cancer
- Alcohol
- Smoking
- Having received radiation that included the breast
- Age at first menstruation
- Past pregnancies
- Not breastfeeding a child
- Late menopause

Obesity

Research has demonstrated that chubby women of any race or ethnicity have an increased risk for developing breast cancer. Unfortunately, studies have found that there is a higher percentage of obesity among black women than among white women. According to the American Cancer Society, more than half (57 percent) of all black women were obese in the United States in 2012 compared to 39 percent of white women.[18]

It is not known exactly *how* obesity may cause breast cancer, although it may be that the excessive weight increases the level of circulating female hormones like estrogen, leading to an elevated risk for breast cancer. If you already have been diagnosed with breast cancer, losing weight is the last thing on your mind. But eventually it's best to lose some weight for your future health if you are overweight or obese.

Knowing that obesity is a risk factor for breast cancer may help your overweight family members and friends to decrease their cancer risk by losing some weight. When possible, prevention is always a good idea. Besides, obesity is also risk a factor for many other diseases in addition to breast cancer, such as type 2 diabetes, hypertension, heart disease and stroke, and other forms of cancer.

It's Genetic: Your Female Family Members Who Had Breast Cancer

Because of the continued secrecy and guilt and shame that still surround breast cancer, you may not know if others in your family had this disease. For this reason, and as recommended earlier, you should ask your mother, your sisters, and your aunts if they ever had breast cancer. Males can also get breast cancer and it also is an important indicator for genetic disease. Tell them that scientists have found there's a genetic risk for breast cancer. If you discover that one or more of your biological relatives had breast cancer, then your risk for this disease is increased. You are not doomed to get breast cancer, but the risk of developing cancer is increased. When I say "biological" relatives, I mean relatives with whom you share a genetic link. So, obviously this excludes nonrelative foster children or adopted children, as well as your partner's side of the family (unless your partner is a relative).

Alcohol Abuse

Abuse of alcohol has been linked to an escalated risk for developing breast cancer and a few other cancers.[19] Daily consumption of 50 grams of alcohol per day increases the risk for breast cancer by 1.5 times.[20] According to the National Institute of Alcohol Abuse and Alcoholism (NIAAA), a standard drink has 14 grams of alcohol, and there are 14 grams of alcohol in 12 ounces of regular beer, 5 ounces of table wine, and a shot of 1.5 ounces of distilled spirits.[21] This means that drinking about 3.5 drinks of any of these items is roughly equivalent to 50 grams of alcohol.

Some researchers have found that even a moderate consumption of alcohol before a woman's first pregnancy significantly increases her risk for breast cancer because alcohol causes changes to the breast. According to Ying Liu and colleagues, "Compared with other organs, [the] breast appears to be more susceptible to carcinogenic effects of alcohol. The risk of breast cancer is significantly increased by 4–15% for light alcohol consumption (≤ 1 drink /day or ≤ 12.5 g/day), which does not significantly increase cancer risk in other organs of women. This raises a clinical and public health concern because nearly half of women of child-bearing age drink alcohol and 15% of drinkers at this age have four or more drinks at a time."[22]

Doctors today consider all alcohol use problems as "alcohol use disorders," and they view these disorders on a continuum of their severity. In the worst case, a person is identified as what was (and often still is) called an alcoholic, or a person whose entire life is centered around the abuse of alcohol and who has a problem with work and family members because of this use. When there are problems that don't rise to the level of alcoholism, but there are clear problems with alcohol, this is still an alcohol use disorder but it may correspond to what was called in the past "alcohol abuse." According to the American Psychiatric Association in its *Diagnostic and Statistical Manual of Mental Disorders* (*DSM-5*), alcohol use disorder is mild, moderate, or severe.[23] A person with a severe alcohol use disorder is equivalent to a person who used to be called an alcoholic, or a person with alcohol dependence. This individual is addicted to alcohol.

In general, black people have a lower rate of alcohol use disorders than whites, although of those blacks who do have this problem, these individuals have a higher rate of developing alcohol-related liver diseases than whites, according to the NIAAA.[24] Excessive alcohol consumption also causes liver disease, and can lead to liver failure and death.

If you think you may have an alcohol use disorder, consult your physician for assistance. Drinking alcohol will not help you fight your breast cancer

---

COULD BLACK HAIR PRODUCTS BE IMPLICATED IN BREAST CANCER?

Some researchers speculate that perhaps very strong hair straighteners and perms for black women could increase the environmental risk for developing breast cancer. Many black women use black hair products. According to Laura Stiel and colleagues in their 2016 article for *Cancer Medicine,* there are three possible mechanisms of an increased breast cancer risk in hair products such as hair relaxers or hair root stimulators, including estrogens used to promote hair growth, phthalates used to perfume the hair products, and parabens used as preservatives.[1] Further research is needed on this subject.

[1]Laura Stiel et al., "A Review of Hair Product Use on Breast Cancer Risk in African American Women," *Cancer Medicine* 5, no. 3 (2016): 597–604.

effectively, and you need to marshal all your mental and physical faculties to be as strong as possible.

Smoking

Smoking is the single most preventable cause of death, according to the surgeon general in the United States.[25] For many years, doctors have known that smoking causes lung cancer and increases the risk for many other forms of cancer, including breast cancer. In a research report of smoking and the risk of breast cancer among black women, based on 1,377 cases in the Black Women's Health Study and published in *Cancer Causes Control* in 2013, Lynn Rosenberg and colleagues found a significant risk for developing breast cancer before menopause among those women who smoked, particularly among black women who started smoking before age 18 and who had experienced 20 or more years of smoking. The strongest link between smoking and breast cancer was found for estrogen-receptor-positive cancer. The risk for breast cancer was the highest among obese women who smoked.[26]

Passive smoking (not smoking oneself, but being around others who smoke) was also found to be a significant risk factor for developing premenopausal breast cancer among the black female subjects.[27] Yet researchers report that about 10 percent of cancer survivors keep smoking as long as 10 years after their initial diagnosis, particularly younger cancer survivors.[28] This is a really, really bad idea.

Smoking causes so many health problems that it's not worth it for any woman to ever start to smoke. Black women are also at risk for developing lung cancer, as discussed in Chapter Nine. If you already smoke, then giving up smoking now is an excellent idea. It can be very tough to stop smoking with a cancer diagnosis hanging over your head. But breast cancer is bad enough. You don't want to also develop lung cancer or other forms of cancer like colorectal cancer that are linked to smoking. (Colorectal cancer is another form of cancer that is worse among the black population.)

Radiation Treatments and X-Rays

Past radiation that included the breast increases the risk for the development of future cancer, and when you receive radiation for breast cancer, the dosages are high, strong enough to kill those cancer cells. I received radiation for my breast cancer the first time it was diagnosed.

Radiation was part of the treatment that I needed to save my life. Then my breast cancer recurred 18 years later. I also developed thyroid cancer, also affecting my neck, which I believe was related to the high doses of radiation to my chest.

Age at First Menstruation

Some research has shown that a younger age at the time of the first menstruation (age 11 or younger) is associated with an increased risk for breast cancer later in life, while an older age (14 years or older) is a protective factor against breast cancer.[29]

Past Pregnancies and Number of Pregnancies/Children

Whether a woman has been pregnant in the past and how old she was at the time of her first pregnancy are also risk factors tied to breast cancer. For example, some researchers have found that three or more pregnancies/births decrease the risk for breast cancer. However, in one study among black women, the researchers found that three or more births were associated with an increased risk of one type of breast cancer (estrogen negative and progesterone negative) but a decreased risk for estrogen-positive and progesterone-positive breast cancer.[30]

Other researchers have found that at least one full-term pregnancy is protective against the *BRCA1* gene.[31]

Some research indicates that having had no children or having a first child after age 30 increases the risk for breast cancer.[32] See Table 1.1 for other risk factors for breast cancer.

Breastfeeding a Child

Some research indicates that breastfeeding a child for at least six months *decreases* the risk for breast cancer, while *not* breastfeeding increases the risk. Breastfeeding is particularly protective against triple-negative cancer in women of childbearing age.[33] Some researchers have stated that black women are less likely to breastfeed their children than white women and this may be one reason for a higher risk of breast cancer in black women. This may be because there are fewer breastfeeding role models in the community. In addition, low income, a lack of personal support, and workplaces that are unsupportive of breastfeeding may also contribute to lower rates of breastfeeding among black women, according to experts seeking to increase the rate of breastfeeding among black women.[34]

Table 1.1   Risk Factors for Breast Cancer in Women

Gynecologic risk factors	• Menstruating at or before age 11
	• Not breastfeeding a child
	• Having no children or having the first child after age 30
	• Late menopause
	• Not having regular gynecologic checkups
	• Not having mammograms (mammograms don't prevent breast cancer but they can detect early and treatable cancers)
Behavioral risk factors	• Smoking
	• Consuming alcohol, even in small amounts
	• Being obese
Genetic factors	• Carrying the *BRCA1* or *BRCA1* gene
	• Having a family member who has had breast cancer (mother, sister, daughter, or father—men also can get breast cancer)
Past medical issues	• Having had breast cancer in the past
Treatment factors	• Having had radiation therapy to the chest (routine chest X-rays for pneumonia, etc., do not count)
Other risk factors	• Being black
	• Being poor
	• Lack of knowledge
	• Fear of health system

Later Menopause

Some researchers have found that a later-than-normal menopause (after age 55 years) increases the risk for breast cancer. This may be because of the greater number of menstrual cycles, although the reasons are yet unknown.[35]

Behavioral or Cultural Factors Linked to Breast Cancer

Again, it's not your fault that you developed breast cancer but you may fit into one or more criteria of people who are more likely than others to end up with this diagnosis. Researchers have some theories about the possible reasons for the disparities in breast cancer among different races and ethnicities, based on research studies. These theories center around the following potential factors among black women:

- Delayed or absent annual gynecologic checkups
- Less access to health care
- Black women get more aggressive tumors than white women
- Poverty
- Denial
- Fear and mistrust of the healthcare system
- Lack of knowledge
- Misguided spirituality
- Other combined factors

Delayed or Absent Gynecologic Checkups

It's important to visit your gynecologist for an annual checkup, especially if you are of childbearing age, 18–45 years old. It doesn't matter whether you want to or even can have children; what matters is your age. Be sure to receive an annual gynecological examination.

If you or your daughter or your friends don't have health insurance or Medicaid, there are federal and state programs available to pay the cost for you to have a mammogram. For example, the National Breast and Cervical Cancer Early Detection Program helps poor and uninsured women obtain clinical breast examinations and mammograms. It's available in every state, based on the Breast and Cervical Cancer Prevention and Treatment Act passed in 2000. One major drawback to this program is that the organization concentrates on screening women aged 40 and older. To find the toll-free number to call in your state and find where you can obtain screening, go to this site: https://nccd.cdc.gov/dcpc_Programs/index.aspx#/1.

I realize, of course, that modern women are extremely busy, and going to an annual doctor's appointment may seem like a waste of time. You may have to find someone to watch the kids, take time off from work, and reschedule other things that seem much more important to you. Don't make this mistake. Schedule that annual checkup!

Less Access to Health Care

The Affordable Healthcare Act was designed to make health care available to all Americans, although there are likely some individuals who still fall through the gap. There are also other issues that make health care harder to access. For example, perhaps you don't have transportation to the doctor's office. Can you take a bus, or get a ride from a friend? Once you have been diagnosed with breast cancer, you must find a way to get to your doctor so that you can obtain treatment. Many cancer centers provide transportation for patients. Please enquire. It's crucial for you to receive treatment. Don't delay. Ask for help when you need it.

Black Women Get More Aggressive Tumors

There's not much that we black women can do about our higher risk for very dangerous tumors of the breast. But it's all the more reason to insist on an annual checkup. Also, if your mother or sister was diagnosed with breast cancer before she was 40 years old, insist on a mammogram in your thirties. You would fight for your children, wouldn't you? Then fight for yourself so you can be alive and available to your children for as long as possible.

Poverty

Black women are more likely to be poor than white women, and this problem continues in the United States despite years of many efforts to improve it. Research indicates that women of higher socioeconomic status and higher levels of education are more likely to obtain a mammogram than are poor women. In a study of 516 women in low-income areas of Alabama, Rupak Chowdhury and colleagues found that low income, low education, and lack of a family doctor were all predictive for not getting a mammogram.[36] In a much larger study of more than 2,000 women of color compared to more than 4,000 women of Anglo-European ancestry,

---

PROTECT YOURSELF FROM X-RAYS WITH A THYROID GUARD

I strongly recommend that *any* woman having X-rays or any type of radiation for any reason whatsoever should be sure to use a *thyroid guard*. When you go to the dentist and the dentist x-rays your mouth, ask for a thyroid guard! This is a little collar that goes over your neck and protects your thyroid from radiation similar to the heavy apron device that everyone uses now to protect the front part of your body.

the researchers found that women living in poor or near-poor neighborhoods in California were disadvantaged compared to the other women, whether the women of color had health insurance or not.[37]

Women who are poor should have access to health care, including gynecological examinations, pap smears, and mammograms. But they may lack access to a car or bus to get to a doctor's appointment. Many cancer centers provide transportation for patients. However, transportation is not the only problem. I personally had to take more than a month off for chemotherapy because it was so debilitating that I could barely stand and could not work. I am not afflicted with poverty; but low-income black women may not be able to afford to take that much time off. The Family and Medical Leave Act does not provide for paid leave. Women need to feed their families. I get that.

I support universal health care because even the successes of Obamacare are not sufficient for many black women—or for poor women of other races or ethnicities.

Denial

Denial of their breast cancer is another common problem among black women as well as women of all races and ethnicities. Nobody wants to think that they could have breast cancer. So, women delay or altogether forget to make an appointment with the gynecologist or to go to get that mammogram or that annual checkup with the gynecologist. And years go by and breast cancer may then develop into a major deadly invader. Black women don't have the luxury of time that individuals of other races have, and consequently, this is yet another reason why we black women should not delay our breast cancer screening.

Fear and Mistrust of the Healthcare System

Some black women are afraid to see their doctors and they are particularly fearful of having tests such as the mammogram. In a study of 29 black low-income women in Chicago, Monica E. Peek and colleagues found that several key common themes arose among the women regarding their negative attitudes about mammogram screening.[38] One issue was prior negative experiences with healthcare providers, such as doctors or mammogram technicians. The women who complained about these issues said that they felt that medical professionals were dismissive or disrespectful to them. In addition, some of the women were afraid that they would be directed to have unnecessary surgery, while others said they were afraid of the doctor.

In a study of 32 black mothers and their daughters by Maghboeba Mosavel and colleagues regarding attitudes toward screening for breast cancer and cervical cancer, the researchers found several key barriers toward getting a mammogram.[39] Nineteen percent of the mothers said that they felt that mammograms were too painful, which was an attitudinal barrier to getting a mammogram, and 16 percent of the women said they were afraid that the mammogram might detect something wrong. Not knowing was apparently perceived as a better choice than knowing if cancer was present in these individuals. This is an attitude I'm fighting against by writing this book. Knowing *is* better. Because when you know your enemy, then you can become armed for battle. Ignorance of cancer is not bliss.

Let me ask you this. Would you rather that your partner or your friends avoid the mammogram or other tests that might show they have cancer? Wouldn't you think it was better for them to know so they could act against that cancer? Think about it. Other people care about you and they want you to stay in the best of health that you can achieve.

Lack of Knowledge

Researchers have found that a lot of the fear about getting a mammogram centered around a lack of information and poor communication between healthcare providers and women. Some research has supported the idea that some doctors are less likely to explain preventive care or treatment to black patients.[40] It's not clear if this is caused by racism or other factors. For example, doctors may assume that a woman already knows why mammograms are needed and what their findings may indicate and, consequently, may fail to explain the purpose and the importance of mammograms to her.

Misguided Spirituality

Women who are religious may believe that if they develop breast cancer, then it must be God's will for it to happen. They believe in prayer and they may be highly skeptical of breast cancer screening and what it could show. I've already discussed my views on this issue, but it's worth saying one more time: I think God wants us to use the cancer doctors that he put on this earth to treat us and hopefully cure us when we're sick.

Other Combined Factors

In an analysis of 18 studies with more than 6,000 black participants, researchers Claire E. L. Jones and colleagues studied factors that created barriers to the early diagnosis of breast cancer among black women. They found that the research showed that the key factors in delaying diagnosis were a lack of knowledge about breast cancer symptoms and risk factors, as well as fear of abandonment by their partners, fear of the identification of an abnormality, fear of treatment for cancer, embarrassment in talking about their symptoms with healthcare professionals, and the stigma and taboo associated with breast cancer.[41] The key word in many of these findings was "fear." Knowledge trumps fear, and that is another reason why my goal is to provide information and education.

My Story

Everyone who has ever had breast cancer has their own story to tell and I'm going to tell you my story. Before I was diagnosed with breast cancer, I had experienced really bad problems with uterine fibroids, another common problem among black women. I wondered if those tumors could be present anywhere else in my body. I asked the doctor for an order for a mammogram and he gave me one. It was around the holidays when I got my mammogram, and I had an extra day off from work. When I was finished, the radiologist decided to take more X-rays and within the next few days I was referred to a surgeon. It was very scary.

Next, I had a biopsy in my doctor's office, and it came back cancerous. The tumor was 3–5 centimeters in size, and my lymph nodes were clear, which was a very good thing. Then we discussed my surgery and whether I should have a lumpectomy or a mastectomy (complete removal of the breast). Like most women, I didn't want to lose my breast, so I chose the lumpectomy at age 39. In hindsight, I wish I had gotten the bilateral mastectomy (removal of both breasts) back then in my younger days—but I didn't.

After my surgery, I had 33 radiation treatments from August through October. Then I started chemotherapy in November and had four cycles of chemotherapy from November to the following February. The chemotherapy put me flat on my back: I couldn't work because I was so weak, so I missed four months of work altogether because it took me a month to recover from the chemo.

About 16 years later, I developed thyroid cancer. Nobody ever said it was caused by my radiation treatments but some studies indicate that radiation can cause thyroid cancer. I already had a low thyroid condition and was taking supplemental thyroid medicine. Then nodules started developing on my thyroid and they showed up on a computerized tomography (CT) scan. I had a biopsy and these nodules were benign. I had regular biopsies up until November 2012, when a biopsy showed abnormal cells. So I had a total thyroidectomy and I take an increased dose of thyroid medication now.

Then in 2014, my breast cancer came back. I had a mammogram and the doctor said those distressing words again, that I needed more pictures. I also had an ultrasound, and there it was—the cancer. I have always checked my breasts for lumps but this one was in front of the scar tissue from the first surgery. I contacted my surgeon and he got me in right away. This was 18 years after the first breast cancer surgery.

I told the doctor that I wanted a bilateral mastectomy and the surgeon agreed. It was a good thing I had both breasts removed because when the pathology report came back, it showed that the other breast had cancer cells too. After the surgery, the pathology report came back and there were cancer cells right on the edge of where the doctor did the surgery. This meant that I had to go back and have the rest of the cancer cells removed. More surgery. Let me tell you, I was not a happy patient. My surgeon had said to me, "Cheryl, you do everything that you can do to fight this cancer and leave the rest up to God. Consider me your guide and I'm going to lead you through this." And he did.

A lot of women get breast implants after mastectomy, and I discuss this option in Chapter Six. But I couldn't do that because there was so little skin left because of the radiation and my skin couldn't expand enough to accommodate implants.

It was the grace of God that led me to every cancer diagnosis. Each time that gentle voice of God set up the situation to find each tumor. I am grateful to the Lord that I was obedient and listened. Before each surgery, I went to the pastors of the church according to the scriptures (James 5:14–16): "Is any sick among you? Let him call for the Elders of the church; and let them pray over him, anointing him with oil in the name of the Lord."

Prayer is good because the Lord can heal anyone, but He also gave us healthcare professionals to help heal the sick. Why not let the healthcare professionals get the victory by witnessing the wonderful works and miracles of the Lord?

I had a friend who was diagnosed with breast cancer before me, and when she went back for her second round of chemotherapy, her blood counts were too low to receive chemo, so she was told to wait until the levels came back up. Sometimes that happens with chemotherapy, which can cause low blood counts and other side effects. But instead of waiting until she recovered and resuming her chemo, my friend took her low blood levels as a sign that it wasn't meant for her to have chemo, and a few years later, the cancer had come back, and she passed on because there were no available treatments for her.

I've talked to a lot of people who knew what they were supposed to do about their cancer, but they did not follow the medical advice they were given. Some of them chose to change their diet and add vitamins and herbs. Sometimes people ask me if the holistic route is the way to go with cancer, and I tell them, "I know many people who've gone that route and they're not here to answer you. They lost their battle with cancer."

I tell everyone they need to get screening mammograms. Some people have even called me the Breast Cancer Checker! That's okay with me because I know people who got a mammogram at my insistence, and they later called me to tell me their mammogram had shown cancer. Otherwise, they never would have known they had cancer. I decided I needed to write a book for black women because many of them don't realize how dangerous breast cancer (and other cancers) is for them and they also don't realize that screening can detect these cancers and can get you treated, and then you go on and live your life.

In the past, a lot of black women died of breast cancer as well as from other types of cancer, and quite often, nobody knew what they died from. It's hard for younger people to believe this, but years ago, black people weren't allowed to go to doctors or hospitals. That's in the past. You *can* get cancer screening now and you *can* get treatment. You are no longer blocked from these options, and that's a very good thing because cancer of any type is nothing to be passive about.

It's your adversary and it's a tough one. But there are good treatments and you need to use them.

Notes

1. Lesley A. Stead et al., "Triple-Negative Breast Cancers Are Increased in Black Women Regardless of Age or Body Mass Index," *Breast Cancer Research* 11, no. 2 (2009), http:breast-cancer-research.com/content/11/1/R18 (accessed May 10, 2016); P. Boyle, "Triple-Negative Breast Cancer: Epidemiological Considerations and Recommendations," *Annals of Oncology* 23, Suppl. 6 (2012): vi7–vi12; Bryan Goldner et al., "Incidence of Inflammatory Breast Cancer in Women, 1992–2009, United States," *Annals of Surgical Oncology* 21, no. 4 (April 2014): 1267–1270; Magdalena L. Plasilova et al., "Features of Triple-Negative Breast Cancer: Analysis of 38,813 Cases from the National Cancer Database," *Medicine*, March 28–29, 2015.

Presented at the Society of Surgical Oncology, Houston, Texas, https://www.ncbi.nlm.nih.gov/pmc/articles/PMC5008562/pdf/medi-95-e4614.pdf (accessed September 16, 2016); Eric C. Dietze et al., "Triple-Negative Breast Cancer in African-American Women: Disparities versus Biology," *Nature Reviews Cancer* 15, no. 4 (2015): 248–254.

2. American Cancer Society, *Breast Cancer*, Atlanta, GA, May 4, 2016, http://www.cancer.org/acs/groups/cid/documents/webcontent/003090-pdf.pdf (accessed September 10, 2016).

3. Monica D'Arcy et al., "Race-Associated Biological Differences among Luminal A Breast Tumors," *Breast Cancer Research and Treatment* 152, no. 2 (2015): 437–448.

4. Foluso D. Ademuywa et al., "United States Breast Cancer Mortality Trends in Young Women according to Race," *Cancer* 121, no. 9 (2015): 1469–1476; Anne Marie McCarthy, "Increasing Disparities in Breast Cancer Mortality from 1979 to 2010 for US Black Women Ages 20 to 49 Years," *American Journal of Public Health* 105, Suppl. 3 (July 2015): S446–S448; Bijou Hunt, Steve Whitman, and Marc S. Hurlbert, "Increasing Black: White Disparities in Breast Cancer Mortality in the 50 Largest Cities in the United States," *Cancer Epidemiology* 38 (2014): 118–123.

5. Foluso D. Ademuywa et al., "United States Breast Cancer Mortality Trends in Young Women according to Race," *Cancer* 121, no. 9 (2015): 1469–1476.

6. Carol E. DeSantis et al., "Breast Cancer Statistics, 2015: Convergence of Incidence Rates between Black and White Women," *CA: A Cancer Journal for Clinicians* 66, no. 1 (January/February 2016): 31–42.

7. Anne Marie McCarthy, "Increasing Disparities in Breast Cancer Mortality from 1979 to 2010 for US Black Women Ages 20 to 49 Years," *American Journal of Public Health* 105, Suppl. 3 (July 2015): S446–S448.

8. Ibid.

9. American Cancer Society, *Breast Cancer*. Atlanta, GA: American Cancer Society, May 4, 2016, http://www.cancer.org/acs/groups/cid/documents/webcontent/003090-pdf.pdf (accessed September 10, 2016).

10. Azadeh Stark et al., "African Ancestry and Higher Prevalence of Triple-Negative Breast Cancer: Findings from an International Study," *Cancer* 116, no. 21 (November 1, 2010): 4926–4932; Edmund M. Der et al., "Triple-Negative Breast Cancer in Ghanaian Women: The Korle Bu Teaching Hospital Experience," *The Breast Journal* 21, no. 6 (2015): 627–633.

11. Tomi Akinyemiju, Swati Sakhuja, and Neomi Vin-Raviv, "Racial and Socio-Economic Disparities in Breast Cancer Hospitalization Outcomes by Insurance Status," *Cancer Epidemiology* 43 (2016): 63–69.

12. Albert Siu, on behalf of the U.S. Preventive Task Force, "Screening for Breast Cancer: U.S. Preventive Task Force Recommendation Statement," *Annals of Internal Medicine* 164, no. 4 (February 16, 2016): 279–296. http://annals.org/aim/article/2480757/screening-breast-cancer-u-s-preventive-services-task-force-recommendation (accessed April 7, 2017).

13. American Cancer Society, "American Cancer Society Guidelines for the Early Detection of Cancer," July 26, 2016, https://www.cancer.org/healthy/find-cancer-early/cancer-screening-guidelines/american-cancer-society-guidelines-for-the-early-detection-of-cancer.html (accessed April 8, 2017).

14. American College of Obstetricians and Gynecologists "ACOG Statement on Breast Cancer Screening Guidelines," January 11, 2016, http://www.acog.org/About-ACOG/News-Room/Statements/2016/ACOG-Statement-on-Breast-Cancer-Screening-Guidelinesm (accessed April 20, 2017).

Some agencies are even *worse*. For example, the U.S. Preventive Services Task force in 2016 recommended making mammogram screening optional until age 50! This would be terrible for black women! https://www.cdc.gov/cancer/breast/pdf/BreastCancerScreeningGuidelines.pdf.

15. P. Boyle, "Triple-Negative Breast Cancer: Epidemiological Considerations and Recommendations," *Annals of Oncology* 23, Suppl. 6 (2012): vi7–vi12; Kathryn C. Amirikia, Paul Mills, Jason Bush, and Lisa A. Newman, "Higher Population-Based Incidence Rates of Triple-Negative Breast Cancer among Young African-American Women," *Cancer* 117, no. 12 (June 15, 2011): 2747–2753; Katrina F. Trivers et al., "The Epidemiology of Triple-Negative Breast Cancer, Including Race," *Cancer Causes Control* 20, no. 7 (September 2009): 1071–1082; Betsy A. Kohler et al., "Annual Report to the Nation on the Status of Cancer, 1975–2011, Featuring Incidence of Breast Cancer Subtypes by Race/Ethnicity, Poverty, and State," *Journal of the National Cancer Institute* 107, no. 6 (June 2015), doi:10.1093/jnci/djv048, https://www.ncbi.nlm.nih.gov/pmc/articles/PMC4603551/ (accessed October 1, 2016).

16. Tuya Pal et al., "A High Frequency of BRCA Mutations in Young Black Women with Breast Cancer Residing in Florida," *Cancer* 121, no. 23 (December 2015): 4173–4180.

17. Ibid.

18. American Cancer Society, *Breast Cancer*, Atlanta, GA: American Cancer Society, May 4, 2016, http://www.cancer.org/acs/groups/cid/documents/webcontent/003090-pdf.pdf (accessed September 10, 2016).

19. Robert Baan et al., "Carcinogenicity of Alcoholic Beverages," *Lancet Oncology* 8, no. 4 (April 2007): 292–293, http://www.thelancet.com/pdfs/journals/lanonc/PIIS1470-2045(07)70099-2.pdf (accessed September 23, 2016).

20. N. Hamajima et al., "Alcohol, Tobacco and Breast Cancer: Collaborative Reanalysis of Individual Data from 53 Epidemiological Studies, Including 58,515 Women without the Disease," *British Journal of Cancer* 87 (2002): 1234–1245.

21. National Institute on Alcohol Abuse and Alcoholism, "What Is a Standard Drink?" undated, https://www.niaaa.nih.gov/alcohol-health/overview-alcohol-consumption/what-standard-drink (accessed September 23, 2016).

22. Ying Liu, Nhi Nguehen, and Graham A. Colditz, "Links between Alcohol Consumption and Breast Cancer: A Look at the Evidence," *Women's Health* 11, no. 1 (2015): 65.

23. American Psychiatric Association, *Diagnostic and Statistical Manual of Mental Disorders, Fifth Edition (DSM-5)* (Washington, DC: American Psychiatric Association, 2013).

24. Karen G. Chartier, Patrice A. C. Vaeth, and Raul Caetano, "Focus on Ethnicity and the Social and Health Harms from Drinking," *Alcohol Research: Current Reviews* 35, no. 2 (2013): 229–237, http://pubs.niaaa.nih.gov/publications/arcr352/229-237.pdf (accessed September 20, 2016).

25. U.S. Department of Health and Human Services, *The Health Consequences of Smoking—50 Years of Progress: A Report of the Surgeon General.* Atlanta, GA: U.S. Department of Health and Human Services, Centers for Disease Control and Prevention, National Center for Chronic Disease Prevention and Health Promotion, Office on Smoking and Health, 2014, http://www.surgeongeneral.gov/library/reports/50-years-of-progress/exec-summary.pdf (accessed September 20, 2016).

26. Lynn Rosenberg et al., "A Prospective Study of Smoking and Breast Cancer Risk among African-American Women." *Cancer Causes Control* 24 (2013): 2207–2215.

27. Ibid.

28. Kimberly D. Miller et al., "Cancer Treatment and Survivorship Statistics, 2016," *CA Cancer Journal Clinics* 66 (2016): 271–289.

29. Julia S. Sisti et al., "Reproductive Factors, Tumor Receptor Status and Contralateral Breast Cancer Risk: Results from the WECARE Study," *SpringerPlus* 4 (2015).

30. Julie R. Palmer et al., "Parity and Lactation in Relation to Estrogen Receptor Negative Breast Cancer in African American Women," *Cancer Epidemiology, Biomarkers & Prevention,* 20, no. 9 (2011): 1883–1891.

31. Angela Toss et al., "The Impact of Reproductive Life on Breast Cancer Risk in Women with Family History or BRCA Mutation," *Oncotarget,* November 17, 2016, https://www.researchgate.net/publication/310765091_The_impact_of_repro ductive_life_on_breast_cancer_risk_in_women_with_family_history_or_BRCA_ mutation (accessed November 29, 2016).

32. American Cancer Society, What Are the Risk Factors for Breast Cancer?" September 13, 2016, http://www.cancer.org/cancer/breastcancer/detailedguide/breast-cancer-risk-factors (accessed November 29, 2016).

33. Christopher I. Li et al., "Reproductive Factors and Risk of Estrogen Receptor Positive, Triple-Negative, and HER2-Neu Overexpressing Breast Cancer among Women 20–44 Years of Age," *Breast Cancer Research and Treatment* 137, no. 2 (2013): 579–587.

34. Angela Johnson et al., "Enhancing Breastfeeding Rates Among African American Women: A Systematic Review of Current Psychosocial Interventions," *Breastfeeding Medicine* 10, no. 1 (2015): 45–62.

35. American Cancer Society, "What Are the Risk Factors for Breast Cancer?" September 13, 2016, http://www.cancer.org/cancer/breastcancer/detailedguide/breast-cancer-risk-factors (accessed November 29, 2016).

36. Rupak Chowdhury et al., "Assessing the Key Attributes of Low Utilization of Mammography Screening and Breast-self Exam among African American Women," *Journal of Cancer* 7, no. 5 (2016), http://www.jcancer.org/v07p0532.htm (accessed August 16, 2016).

37. Sundus Haji-Jama et al., "Disparities among Minority Women with Breast Cancer Living in Impoverished Areas of California," *Cancer Control* 23, no. 2 (April 2016): 157–162.

38. Monica, E. Peek, Judith V. Sayad, and Ronald Markwardt, "Fear, Fatalism and Breast Cancer Screening in Low-Income African-American Women: The Role of Clinicians and the Health Care System," *Journal of General Internal Medicine* 23, no. 11 (2008): 1847–1853.

39. Maghboeba Mosavel et al., "Communication Strategies to Reduce Cancer Disparities: Insights from African-American Mother-Daughter Dyads," *Family Sys Health* 33, no. 4 (December 2015): 400–404.

40. Oliver, M. Norman, et al., "Time Use in Clinical Encounters: Are African-American Patients Treated Differently?" *Journal of the National Medical Association* 93, no. 10 (2001): 380–385; Monica, E. Peek, Judith V. Sayad, and Ronald Markwardt, "Fear, Fatalism and Breast Cancer Screening in Low-Income African-American Women: The Role of Clinicians and the Health Care System," *Journal of General Internal Medicine* 23, no. 11 (2008): 1847–1853.

41. Claire E. L. Jones et al., "A Systematic Review of Barriers to Early Presentation and Diagnosis with Breast Cancer among Black Women," *BMJ Open* (2014), http://bmjopen.bmj.com/content/4/2/e004076.full.pdf+html (accessed August 6, 2016).

CHAPTER TWO

Dealing with Common Emotions and Talking to Others

The first thought I had when I received my breast cancer diagnosis was, "I'm going to die." Then the second thought was, "Who will take care of my children?"

—A black woman diagnosed with breast cancer

So many different and powerful emotions overwhelm the woman who has just been diagnosed with breast cancer. Black women are like women of other races and ethnicities in terms of their many fears, such as the fear of death, the fear for what will happen to their children, and the fear of the loss of their femininity. Panic, anxiety, sadness, depression, and fear are also common emotions that flood into the brain of the woman who has just been diagnosed with breast cancer. These emotions may wane and then may come back again periodically because breast cancer is such a devastating diagnosis. Some black women with breast cancer are sad to the point of being clinically depressed, which means that they need treatment also for their depression. High risk factors for depression among black women include a diagnosis with triple negative cancer and chronic stress levels.[1]

Black women with breast cancer may have extra emotional differences from women of other races in that some black women may be more mistrustful of physicians and more reticent about telling other people that they have been diagnosed with cancer. It's hard to know for sure because there are so few studies of black women with breast cancer, and often these studies concentrate on low-income women only.

Yet there are middle-class and wealthy black women who develop breast cancer too. Some research indicates that more educated women are less fearful of breast cancer than poorly educated women, so maybe black women of a higher socioeconomic status are stronger than poor women. But they're still women, no matter how much money is in their bank account, and breast cancer is a frightening diagnosis for any woman.

In Chapter One, I talked briefly about some of the key fears preventing black women from taking needed action to obtain a diagnosis of their breast cancer in the first place, such as fear of the discovery of cancer, fear of partner abandonment, embarrassment at dealing with healthcare professionals, and other fears. In this chapter, I talk about fears and other emotional reactions when a cancer diagnosis is a reality for a woman.

This chapter covers the basic fears and concerns experienced by black women with breast cancer and also discusses how to talk to others about your cancer diagnosis. In addition, I talk about how joining a support group of women with breast cancer may help you considerably in dealing with your fears and anxieties. Last, I cover the aggravating comments that people sometimes make to women who have breast cancer, and offer you suggestions on how to respond.

Common Emotional Reactions to a Breast Cancer Diagnosis

The most common emotional reactions to a breast cancer diagnosis are the following:

- Fear of death
- Fear of loss of femininity
- Anger
- Anxiety and panic
- Fear of what will happen to your children
- Fear of rejection by others
- Depression
- Cancer-related posttraumatic stress
- Feelings of helplessness
- Feeling betrayed by your own body
- Shame and embarrassment
- Feeling a loss of control

The Fear of Death

When receiving a breast cancer diagnosis, the fear of death is nearly a universal emotion among women. Of course women realize that they are not immortal beings, but the reality is that most people don't think about their own deaths very much, if at all. You just go about your day and make your plans, and do the best you can, even though you know you're mortal and will someday die. It just seems that death is a long way off. However, a diagnosis of cancer brings the idea of your death into very sharp focus.

Some research has shown that some black women believe that a diagnosis of breast cancer at any stage is equivalent to a death sentence, and they don't realize that the early diagnosis and treatment of breast cancer bring the best likelihood of cure and continued life. And even if you cannot be cured, early treatment brings the best prognosis for an extended life. When you learn that you have breast cancer, the worst thing to do is to do nothing.

Fear of Loss of Femininity

The breast is a big deal in the United States. Big-breasted women are proud of (or sometimes embarrassed by) their figure, and often the first part of the body men look at is not the eyes or the legs, but the breasts. Some men brag that they are "boob men." As a result, some healthy small-breasted women undergo cosmetic surgery to get breast implants. In our culture, the breast is an important part of sexuality and sex. It's also linked to motherhood and nurturing, although many women forego breastfeeding. So it's understandable that considering the loss of all or even a part of a breast because of breast cancer is a very scary idea. It's not like having your appendix out. Nobody ever sees or cares about your appendix unless you need emergency surgery, and it's only the doctor who sees it. In contrast, with the removal of all or part of the breast, it's like taking away a female part, even if surgery means a lumpectomy, rather than a complete removal of the breast.

Many women fear that their spouses or significant others will no longer want to have sex with them after surgery for breast cancer, and that they will seek out other sexual partners who do have breasts and haven't had cancer. They also fear that their partner may leave them. Because of these multiple fears, some women may decide to avoid having breast cancer screening altogether. They'd rather not know than have a mammogram.

I'm here to tell you that this is a very bad idea. The mammogram takes only a few minutes, but the information it yields can mean the difference between life and death. Choose life.

I don't know if the fear of the loss of the breast is greater in black women than in women of other races or ethnicities, but I suspect that it may be. Call it a gut feeling.

Anger

Anger, or even the intensified feeling of rage, is another common emotional reaction to receiving a diagnosis of breast cancer. You may say to yourself, "*Why* did this have to happen to me? *How* could this have happened to me? What did I ever do to deserve such a terrible thing as breast cancer? It isn't fair!" You may feel like a person who is suffering a great injustice. You might even be angry with God, as presumptuous as that sounds. I too asked God, "Why me?" When I was going through radiation treatment and I witnessed small children who had to be sedated to have the same radiation treatment that I was having, that small voice from God said, "Why not you?"

I believe that breast cancer just happens, and often you never know why it happens. It might be because of the genes in your body or it could be a combination of other factors, but that information may never be revealed to you because the doctors don't know why you got breast cancer either. Understand that anger is a common reaction to a breast cancer diagnosis. Mobilize the energy from that anger to help you learn everything you can about your diagnosis and treatment.

Anxiety and Panic

When something really distressing happens to most people, they feel a basic "fight or flight" natural urge, which means that either they want to run away or they feel frozen in place. With breast cancer, the fight or flight reaction often translates to severe anxiety and even panic. You can't run away from your own body, but you wish you could, when you have a cancer diagnosis hanging over your head. Anxiety can also cause you to think of the worst possible things that could ever happen to you with a breast cancer diagnosis, like dying tomorrow or even today. Or it could make you imagine that you will have terrible and unbearable pain or that nobody will help you or care about you anymore. Many kinds of thoughts may swirl around in the mind of the anxious person. Researchers call it "catastrophizing," because the anxious mind often defaults to the worst possible causes imaginable.

Let's face it; most women who are diagnosed with breast cancer likely have some pretty dark thoughts when they first learn about their diagnosis. The key is to pull yourself out of this anxious state so you can attend to learning what your treatment options are and then proceeding forth through those treatments. How can you do that?

One way is by saying to yourself, in your mind, "I will be okay, whatever happens." Imagine saying this to yourself in a confident voice, the kind of voice you use when you know exactly what you are doing. Drown out the anxious thoughts with this strong and confident voice. This doesn't sound like it'll work, but it actually does help quite a lot for many situations. Try it.

Another way to overcome anxiety is to take slow, deep breaths and calm your body down. It's harder to think anxious thoughts when you are sitting or lying down and breathing deeply and calmly.

It's also important to have confidence in your doctor. In a study of 82 black women with breast cancer by Vanessa B. Sheppard and colleagues, published in *Psychooncology* in 2014,[2] the researchers found that women with high levels of medical mistrust were significantly more prone to suffer from anxiety or depression than women without this mistrust. In this study, the researchers found that 25 percent of the subjects had clinical or borderline levels of anxiety, while 21 percent had high or borderline levels of depression. Together, a third of the subjects had anxiety or depression that was clinically significant or borderline. Sheppard et al. also found that the younger patients with breast cancer were more likely to experience distress in the form of anxiety or depression.[3] Since black women are more likely to be diagnosed with breast cancer at younger ages than women of other races or ethnicities, this is an important finding.

The bottom line is that you may not be able to avoid anxiety altogether, but if you are genuinely distrustful of your physician, it might be a good idea to get a second or even a third opinion. Maybe your body is telling you something and you need to listen. Or maybe you're being very anxious for no real reason. Talking to other doctors may greatly ease your mind about your diagnosis and treatment.

In some cases, you may need to take a low dose of an anti-anxiety medication or an antidepressant, to better cope with severe symptoms of anxiety or depression.

IF YOU ARE UNSURE ABOUT YOUR ONCOLOGIST

If you mistrust (are leery of) or distrust (do not trust) your cancer doctor, ask yourself the following questions:

- Is it this particular doctor that you have qualms about? Or would any cancer doctor be someone you might fear? Maybe there's something about the doctor him- or herself that you don't like. But maybe it's cancer itself that is scaring you, rather than the doctor, who was the person who first told you about your cancer. Your gut level knows the answer to this question.

- Make a list of all the questions you have about your cancer or your treatment that most trouble you. Then make an appointment to ask the doctor your questions. If he or she doesn't provide answers that you understand, ask for clarification. Yes, doctors are busy. But they should be willing to provide short answers or at least refer you to another person who has the answers.

- Ask yourself that if this doctor were a pediatrician or a general practitioner, would you feel okay with him or her? Is the problem with him or her or with the specialty of oncology?

- Ask the doctor approximately how many patients with breast cancer he has treated. He or she can't give you any names, but can give you numbers. You want an experienced doctor. You don't want him or her learning on you. So, if the doctor has treated less than 10 patients with breast cancer, it may be better for you to see a more experienced oncologist. Note: You may wish to consult with a physician who subspecializes in breast cancer and is located at a National Cancer Institute–designated cancer center. Go to this site for more information: http://www.cancer.net/navigating-cancer-care/cancer-basics/cancer-care-team/find-nci-designated-cancer-center.

If you still don't feel right about the doctor, even after he or she has answered all your questions in what seems to be a reasonable way, then tell the doctor in a respectful tone that you would like to get a second opinion, because this is your life, after all. The doctor won't mind. If he or she *does* mind, then that doctor is not the right doctor for you.

Fear of What Will Happen to Your Children

Mothers who are diagnosed with breast cancer almost automatically worry about who will care for their young or adolescent children if the cancer kills them. Many women today are single mothers, and they may frantically think about whether their siblings or their mom could raise the kids if the worst happens. When you have just received a cancer diagnosis, this fear is premature, but it still comes to mind anyway. Calm down and regroup. The best person to raise your kids is you, so work on finding out what treatment is needed and pursue that path. Of course, it's always good to have a backup plan as well. Life throws us lots of curves and you never know what's going to happen next.

Fear of Rejection by Others

Breast cancer isn't "catching," but you might think that it was based on the fears of some women who have been diagnosed with this disease. They may be afraid to tell their friends or even their partners about the diagnosis.

Another kind is the fear that you will become like "damaged goods" if your treatment includes surgery. One breast cancer survivor said, "I didn't tell anyone I had breast cancer. I finally told my boyfriend the night before surgery. I was afraid and embarrassed and didn't want anyone to know."

I'm sorry to report that some other people may feel this way—that a woman with breast cancer is somehow damaged and no longer fully a female. It's a terrible thing to have to report this, but the reality is that other people don't always react the way we wish they did or the way that they should react. It's also true that you also can't know ahead of time how people will react. Your girlfriend whom you've known forever and who you were sure would be supportive may instead distance herself from you, while others who you never thought would be kind or understanding will far exceed your expectations.

Sadness or Depression

Extreme sadness or even clinical depression frequently is a problem for the woman diagnosed with breast cancer, according to *Psycho-Oncology*,[4] a medical book that concentrates on the feelings that people experience when they learn that they have cancer. If the sadness or depression becomes too overwhelming and difficult to cope with, be sure to tell your doctor. She may recommend therapy and/or antidepressants. Another way to battle depression is to gain emotional support from others in a similar situation. There are many support groups and some should be available in your area. Many groups are also found online, and there are lists of groups in Appendix A of this book. It only makes sense that you need extra emotional support now, but researchers have also verified that, for many individuals, their feelings of sadness or hopelessness decreased with perceived levels of favorable emotional support received from others.

Remember, if you are diagnosed with breast cancer, your attitude is an important percentage of your cure, mentally. Having a good attitude will assist you greatly with your treatment plan. Be ready for the cancer battle and surround yourself with family and friends with the same attitude.

Cancer-Related Posttraumatic Stress

A cancer diagnosis and the continued stress from cancer can lead to a cancer-related posttraumatic stress, according to the National Cancer Institute, which defines this problem as a condition that develops in some people who are diagnosed with cancer. It is characterized by such symptoms as having trouble sleeping and experiencing frightening thoughts, feeling overexcited or distracted, losing interest in daily activities, and feeling all alone. Feelings of shock, fear, and horror may also occur. These symptoms may occur at any time after diagnosis, and are treated with counseling, relaxation therapy, and attendance at support groups with individuals facing the same or similar problem.[5] Anti-anxiety medications and other drugs may also help individuals suffering from cancer-related posttraumatic stress.

It's very important to communicate with your doctors and the clinical team if you have cancer-related posttraumatic stress. They will want to help you. You also need to know that there is no shame in seeing a psychologist or psychiatrist when you need help.

Feelings of Helplessness

Normally you may be a very confident and happy person, but a cancer diagnosis can trigger feelings of helplessness and indecision in the smartest and most capable of women. Without obtaining information on cancer in general, and your type of cancer in particular, you are flying blind and you need to know such information. What you may not realize, however, is that the information is out there and it's available to you. Some information is available through your doctor. A lot of information is available from his nurse and also from other cancer patients. They probably won't have the specific type of breast cancer that you have. But they do know what it feels like to be told you have breast cancer. It's not a pity party to talk with such people. Instead, it helps quite a lot.

Continued feelings of helplessness may morph into depression, already discussed in this chapter. Then it's time to obtain professional help.

Be Careful about What You Believe from the Internet

Note that there is also a great deal of information on the Internet, but much of it is not useful and some of it is even harmful. For example, some websites or individuals may urge you to try the latest supplement or other unproven remedy that they say will "cure" you. Be sure that the information has been vetted by a physician before you accept it as factual. And then check it out with your own oncologist. Just because something is on the Internet doesn't mean it's true.

Feeling Betrayed by Your Own Body

Another common emotion for a woman with breast cancer is to feel like your own body has betrayed you. Maybe you've never smoked and you drink little or no alcohol, and perhaps you've also kept reasonably fit. And the thanks you get for that is your body gets breast cancer. It hardly seems fair. Breast cancer is definitely not fair for any woman, whether she's in good physical shape or not, but it happens anyway. Keep in mind that your body is trying to fight off cancer as best as it can, and you need to do whatever is required to help your body get rid of that cancer. Your body is not your adversary. Your breast is not your adversary either. It is cancer that is your enemy.

Shame and Embarrassment

Some women feel ashamed and embarrassed by their body when they have breast cancer, and these feelings can become intensified if the woman needs surgery. The lumpectomy (removal of the tumor only) may engender less shame and embarrassment than the mastectomy (total removal of one or both breasts), but sometimes mastectomy is needed to get rid of all the cancer and to save your life. Even when women have breast reconstruction after surgery, sometimes they may feel somewhat dissociated from their own body at first. They may also worry that their significant others will no longer find them attractive or even that they will be repulsed by their body. These are all common fears. However, they are definitely not good reasons to forego treatment, as some women do. Again, remember that cosmetic surgery for breast augmentation is very popular among women today of all ages. If you must have a mastectomy, your cosmetic (reconstruction) surgery likely will be covered by insurance and could also come with a bonus abdominoplasty (tummy tuck), a procedure that is necessary to reconstruct your new breast.

Deciding to Move Forward and Get Treatment

You're not going to resolve all your fears, anxieties, sadness, worry about what will happen to the kids, and your other emotions by the time that you will need to start treatment. Often treatment is started immediately when you may barely feel ready to get started. Yet time is not on your side. It's also true that concerns and fears will pop up now and again because this is a very scary time. You may feel like, well, I'm glad that's over, and you think you've mastered your anxiety and sadness, and then for some reason or no reason, there you are, feeling sad or anxious again. Consequently, it's a mistake to delay treatment until you feel that you are completely and 100 percent ready to take on cancer. Cancer has already taken you on. You need to fight back. I will tell you how, throughout this book.

Communicating Well with Your Oncologist

By the time you need to see an oncologist, you've probably seen many doctors, such as a gynecologist, a general practitioner, and maybe a few other doctors. And you've also been talking with people all your life, so you already know how to communicate, right? Well, maybe it would help anyway to have a few pointers in dealing with your doctor, since your time with this person who is very important to your life is limited and you need to get the most benefit out of it. For this reason, I'm including a section on effectively communicating with your doctor.

Thinking about the Past

First I want to take a little detour, and mention here that for many black women, in the not-so-distant past, there have been good reasons to be fearful of doctors, seek to avoid them, and even refuse treatments because of that fear—and these reasons occurred within my lifetime and probably in yours as well. For example, as recently as the late twentieth century, some states involuntarily sterilized black women (and a few white women) who were deemed by others to be unfit to have children. Often they didn't even tell these women what had happened to them, and when the women were unable to have children later, their gynecologist had to break the terrible news to them.

In the worst case that I have read about, a teenage girl in North Carolina was raped and became pregnant in 1967. Right after she had her baby, the state sterilized her, after having labeled her as "feebleminded" and "promiscuous." When she discovered what happened to her later on, she felt like she had been raped two times: once by her assailant and a second time by the state of North Carolina. (North Carolina was not alone in these heinous practices.) North Carolina stopped sterilizing black women in 1977 when it disbanded its eugenics board, the group that decided women's fates, but the law upholding this program was on the books until 2003.[6] This is a very hard story to read about, and I am not bringing this subject up now to impede your communication. It's the opposite. I'm bringing it up because I understand this fear and I want to help you overcome it. Knowledge is power. We black women were denied both knowledge and power in the recent past. No more. That's why it's important to communicate well with your oncologist and other doctors and to ask questions and get answers.

Make a List of Questions Beforehand

Before you even see the doctor, prepare a list of questions and then rank them in order of importance. For example, if you have eight questions, put the most important ones as Numbers 1–4, with the first question as the most important one. The reason for this is if you list the questions in random order, then if time runs short with the doctor, you may not have enough time to learn about the issue that is most pressing to you. Make that Question Number 1. Try to limit your questions to under 7–8, if possible. Throughout this book, I list questions to ask about different forms of therapy, but they don't all need to be asked in one meeting, or "encounter." (Doctors refer to their appointments with you as "encounters"—largely for insurance purposes—which make them sound rather hostile, but they should not be!)

Listen to the Answers

This section may sound silly. Of course, you *listen* to the answers; that's why you asked the question! And yet many people do not really listen, in part because most people think faster than other people can talk—even when the doctor's the one who's talking. So, the mind starts to wander off, and while the doctor is talking on and on, you might wonder what to make for dinner or think about how your feet hurt, and why hasn't your mother called you back today. By the time you get back to the doctor in front of you, you could have totally lost the whole thread of the conversation. To prevent that from happening, think these thoughts as the doctor responds to your question. These are the kind of questions reporters think when they are interviewing people and they work well for others too:

- *What* is the doctor recommending?
- Does it sound like things are going to get worse, stay the same, or get better?
- Is there some time frame during which whatever the doctor is talking about should happen in? Like next week, next month, or some other period of time?
- *Why* is this going to happen?
- *Where* will it happen? In the hospital? An outpatient facility? Or some-place else?
- *Who* is going to provide the recommended action? The doctor? Someone else?
- What is the most important thing to know about your breast cancer? You can tell because the doctor will emphasize a point with his voice or ges-tures. You can also verify by asking the doctor, "Doctor, is (whatever the key point is) the most important thing I need to know about breast cancer?"

Summarize Back What You Think the Doctor Said

When the doctor finishes his answer, tell him or her what you think was just said. For example, "Doctor Brainiac, I think what you're saying is that I will need surgery first, and then radiation therapy. You'll do the surgery but someone else will manage the radiation. Also, you think I have a good chance for a cure." If you're wrong, the doctor will tell you the right information, such as, "Patient X, you got it partly right, you *do* have a good chance for a cure, and you *do* need surgery first, but what I want is for surgery to be followed by chemotherapy because _____."

Stand Your Ground and Don't Be Afraid of the Doctor

If the doctor says he has no time for questions (which he/she should not say!), then say you'll need an appointment when you can get answers to your questions because you need information on which to base your medical decisions. That will usually get the response you want from the doctor, and she will then agree to hear and respond to your questions.

Often the doctor will say that he or she only has five minutes or ten minutes. That's fine, ask your Question Number 1.

Many women are afraid of doctors; trust me, I know this. I know of women who finally worked up their courage to see a doctor about a medical problem, and then the doctor was mean or dismissive, so the women just gave up altogether and walked out of that office and away from any medical treatment at all. Sometimes these actions are cultural and trust issues, because some of us have been reminded of the days when our human rights were violated and doctors experimented on blacks without their knowledge. We fear what the doctor may advise, so we will either don't go to the doctor or walk away without responding, especially if we don't feel comfortable with the doctor.

But don't you walk away! This is your body, this is breast cancer, and you're important. I don't care how much education the doctor has or how many letters go after his or her name. You need information so you can make good choices about your body and your life. Stand your ground. Ask your questions. You don't have to be nasty. Be polite and respectful, but also be assertive. You could say, "Doctor Brainiac, I feel like you are being dismissive to me and not treating me nicely, like I'm not important. But I really need this information from you." If the doctor still isn't helpful—and most *will* be helpful—then you need to see a different doctor.

Bring Someone with You, at Least for the First Few Visits

It's extremely hard to listen well to the doctor describing your diagnosis and planned treatment, yet it's also crucial that you understand what the doctor is telling you. For this reason, it's a good idea to bring a family member or a friend with you. Tell your family member or friend that you don't just want moral support; you want another pair of listening ears. You might even wish to tape-record the doctor if she is okay with that, so you can play the tape back later on to refresh your memory.

Take Simple Notes

If the doctor tells you about things you should do or should not do, it's good to reinforce that information by taking simple notes. Notes are also good for any other information that the doctor says is important. Complete sentences are not required but print or write neatly—you don't want to look at what you wrote later and be unable to decipher your own handwriting. As in a previous example, you could write, "Surgery first, then chemo" to help you remember. You might think that anybody would remember something like this, but you would be wrong! People can forget key information if they don't work at remembering.

Ask the Doctor for Handouts

Presumably the doctor won't give you literature handouts that have any information he is opposed to, so if the physician or his staff give you printouts or brochures, this information will reflect the doctor's views. This literature may also go into more depth and answer other questions that you haven't thought of yet. Reading brochures or handouts can also help you remember the information better.

Telling Your Spouse or Significant Other

There's no easy way to tell your spouse or significant other that you have breast cancer. But you can break it to the other person by saying first that you have something very important and upsetting to say. This will center the concentration on you, so that the other person won't be distracted by the television, the computer, or whatever's going on in his or her head now. The person may worry that you're going to say that you want to break up, so you could also say that it's a problem with your body that you want to talk about.

Many women blurt out the diagnosis to the people who care about them, because they feel like they can no longer hold that information inside anymore. Others are far more reticent about telling other people about cancer and they even hide that information. I think it's a good idea to tell the people that you care about that you carry this emotional burden of having breast cancer. I've provided a sample conversation next in this chapter to help you.

Here is a sample conversation between Shayla and Jamal, when she tells him about her breast cancer diagnosis. It's not meant to be the exact way that you should explain having cancer but instead it is to show how one woman and one man handled the information.

Shayla: Jamal, listen to me. I have something very important to tell you. Important in a bad way.

Jamal: What?

Shayla: Turn off the television, please. This is really important. (She starts crying.)

(Jamal turns off the TV.)

Jamal (looking upset):	What's going on? Are you breaking up with me?
Shayla:	No, it's not that. Not at all. It's my health.
Jamal:	What, are you dying? (He laughs, and then stops laughing when he sees her face.)
Shayla:	No, I'm not dying. But I just found out that I have breast cancer. It's early stage and I can get treated.
Jamal:	But you're too young to get that! That's an old lady disease! You're only forty years old!
Shayla:	I know but I still have it. Black women sometimes get it younger. I definitely have it. I had a mammogram and then some tests, and it's for sure cancer.
Jamal (who starts crying himself):	What are we going to do! This is terrible! I can't believe this! You're such a good woman! This is so wrong!
Shayla:	I need your help. I'm very scared. I need you to try to be strong.
Jamal:	I will try, Shay! But I don't know how to help you!
Shayla:	Just keep loving me and don't ever stop.
Jamal:	I can do that! (The two hug each other.)

Telling or Not Telling People in Your Family

Maybe you're afraid that, if you tell others in your family like your sister, mother, aunt, or cousins that you have breast cancer, they will treat you differently. You may be concerned that others will act like you are a victim and/or a person who is doomed to die right away or in a few years. Maybe you don't want to be an object of pity because you're a proud woman. These views are understandable.

But keep in mind that when you do tell others about your cancer diagnosis, along with all the nonsensical things people may say to you (as discussed later in this chapter), they may also provide you with comfort, caring, and love. It makes sense that women with breast cancer who have the caring support of other people are less likely to be distressed than women who keep the diagnosis all to themselves.

Telling Your Friends and Coworkers

Some people tell certain select family members about their breast cancer but they don't tell their friends or coworkers. This is normal and okay.

You may want to tell just your close friends and the necessary supervisors at work. It is totally up to you. The problem is, others are likely to notice that you are upset and not feeling well. You don't have to tell them but if you don't, they may feel like they must have upset or offended you or that you don't like them anymore. You could say that you have cancer and you don't want to talk about it, but people will then wonder what kind of cancer you have—it's a normal reaction. Let them wonder.

If you want to limit the amount of information you provide to others, you could say that you have breast cancer (or cancer) and that you just don't want to talk about it. You're working on getting treated and you hope everything will get resolved positively. Some people will push for more information, but if you don't want to divulge more, you don't have to. You probably will need to tell the human resources people at your company about your problem, because you'll need extra time off for doctor visits, treatments, and recovery.

Talking with Members of the Clergy

Some black women are strongly religious, and the first person they may consult after receiving a breast cancer diagnosis is their pastor. Most members of the clergy have ministered to people with a cancer diagnosis, and many encourage these individuals to seek treatment.

In one case reported in the *New York Times* in 2013,[7] a black woman was given a breast cancer diagnosis, and her very next act was to go straight to a funeral parlor to plan her funeral and select a casket. When the funeral director heard that the woman was planning her own funeral, he and his wife urged this lady to go see her doctor and work together to make a treatment plan. Instead, she went to see her pastor first. The minister argued with her about seeking treatment until she finally agreed with him that she would consult a physician. She received treatment and apparently is doing well.

Support Groups Can Help Considerably

There are numerous support groups for women with breast cancer. The American Cancer Society chapters or local groups can help match you with another woman who had breast cancer similar to your diagnosis and who understands how you feel. She may not be a black woman, but for the purposes of cancer, you are "sisters" under the skin. You'll be paired with a woman who has come to terms with her cancer, and, believe it or not, someday you will likely wish to help another woman who has been diagnosed with breast cancer.

There are also numerous support groups online for women with breast cancer. There are groups for all women and there are groups for black women. Some examples are the Sisters Network (www.sistersnetworkinc .org), the African American Breast Cancer Alliance (http://aabcainc.org/), and the Living beyond Breast Cancer group (http://www.lbbc.org/african-american), but there are many more groups. Some key groups are listed in Appendix A at the end of this book. The American Cancer Society offers support groups for people of all races and ethnicities.

With online groups, you can read the stories of others after you join the group (and sometimes before), and when you feel comfortable, you may wish to add a question or a comment. Keep in mind, however, that often the people providing information on such groups are not doctors. Always verify information with your own doctor.

Every patient is different when it comes to treatment outcomes to therapy. For example, one person may report a difficult (or easy) time with chemotherapy, yet your experience may be very different. It's also important to understand that prognoses (expected outcomes with treatment) vary considerably, even among people in the same cancer stage. These are reasons why it's crucial to talk to your doctor when you have questions or concerns.

Dealing with Common Annoying Comments People May Make

Many women who have had cancer have said that sometimes other people have made the most annoying and truly upsetting comments to them. This is unfortunate, but it happens. The person may be ignorant or perhaps could be mean-spirited. Or maybe it was a comment that was blurted out without thinking. When people say annoying things, often, later on you think to yourself of what you should have said, but it's too late by then. To help you with that problem, I've created a table to discuss at least a few of the common annoying and nonhelpful things that people often blurt out to women who have breast cancer, and I've also offered my own suggested responses. But I'm sure you could also come up with some good ones of your own!

As you can see from the table, the responses I've offered you as options to make to those ignorant or even mean comments that others may make to you are reasonable and rational. Of course, it's not always easy to be nice when people say awful or stupid things to you about your upsetting cancer diagnosis. Sometimes you may blurt out a retorting comment that

Table 2.1 Annoying comments and what you can say back

Comment	Possible Responses
Are you going to die?	Everyone dies. But if you mean is cancer going to kill me, I hope not. I'm working with my doctor.
My aunt had that and she is no longer with us.	Every case of cancer is different. I'm sorry to hear about your aunt's passing.
Will you still feel like a woman without your breasts?	Not everyone with breast cancer loses their breasts. But I won't suddenly become a man if I need a mastectomy.
Why did you get cancer?	I don't know why. Black women have a higher risk for breast cancer than other women, for unknown reasons.
What did you do wrong to get cancer?	I didn't do anything wrong. Cancer is a medical problem that can affect any women, irrespective of race or age.
You probably got cancer because you were not close enough to God.	How would you know that? Do you know all of my personal time I spend with God every day?
Did you pray enough and go to church every Sunday?	I do pray and go to church frequently. I don't believe that God punishes people by giving them cancer if they miss a church service.
You must have had sex with too many men.	That's a pretty mean thing to say, and it's also not true. Loose women don't get breast cancer more than nice women.
Did you abuse illegal drugs?	Of course I didn't abuse drugs. Even if I had, drug abuse has nothing to do with getting breast cancer.
If you eat a lot of fruit and vegetables, that will help get rid of the cancer.	Once a person has cancer, only treatment gets rid of it unless God heals me. This way we can all rejoice in the miracle and the oncologist will be there to witness the results.
You should go on a special high-fiber diet to cure your cancer.	Once a person has cancer, only treatment gets rid of it unless God heals me. This way we can all rejoice in the miracle and the oncologist will be there to witness the results.
You should do all those things you always wanted to do, just in case.	Just in case I die, you mean? Right now, I'm working to get rid of the cancer.
Who will raise your children?	I plan on raising my own children, if at all possible. If not, I'll make a plan for them.

is equally mean or even worse than what the other person has said to you. If you do, it's okay; you are human. Apologize and move on.

Notes

1. Claudia M. Davis et al., "Biopsychosocial Predictors of Psychological Functioning among African American Breast Cancer Survivors," *Journal of Psychosocial Oncology* 32 (2014): 493–516.

2. Vanessa Sheppard et al., "The Importance of Contextual Factors and Age in Association with Anxiety and Depression in Black Breast Cancer Patients," *Psychooncology* 23, no. 2 (2014): 143–150.

3. Ibid.

4. Julia H. Rowland and Mary Jane Massie, "Breast Cancer," in *Psycho-Oncology, Second Edition,* ed. Jimmie C. Holland et al. (New York: Oxford University Press, 2010), 177–186.

5. National Cancer Institute, *NCI Dictionary of Cancer Terms*, http://www.cancer.gov/publications/dictionaries/cancer-terms (accessed August 8, 2016).

6. Michelle Kessel and Jessica Hopper, "Victims Speak Out about North Carolina Sterilization Program, Which Targeted Women, Young Girls and Blacks," November 7, 2011, http://rockcenter.nbcnews.com/_news/2011/11/07/8640744-victims-speak-out-about-north-carolina-sterilization-program-which-targeted-women-young-girls-and-blacks (accessed September 23, 2016).

7. Tara Parker Pope, "Tackling a Racial Gap in Breast Cancer Survival," *New York Times*, December 20, 2013, http://www.nytimes.com/2013/12/20/health/tackling-a-racial-gap-in-breast-cancer-survival.html?_r=0 (accessed September 23, 2016).

CHAPTER THREE

Types of Breast Cancer
Black Women May Develop

Hearing that you have breast cancer is very scary today, just as it was 25 years ago. But in many ways, breast cancer is also very different from how it was diagnosed and treated in the past, when doctors knew so much less back then than they know now. For example, now every breast cancer tumor is molecularly genetically analyzed (or should be!) to help doctors determine the best treatment for each woman. In addition, some women with breast cancer also receive further genetic analysis to determine if they may carry genetic mutations that could increase their risks for developing breast cancer or for suffering a recurrence of the disease. Hopefully, in another 25 years, advances in breast cancer will be so considerable that this much-feared diagnosis will be perceived as only a minor inconvenience that is easily diagnosed and treated. Sadly, we're not at that point yet.

The types of breast cancer that black women are diagnosed with are the same types as white women or women of other races or ethnicities may develop. However, some types of breast cancer, particularly inflammatory breast cancer (IBC) and triple-negative breast cancer, are much more commonly found among black women.[1] In addition, often breast cancer is more advanced and serious when it is diagnosed in black women. This chapter covers the key types of breast cancers and also describes the types of breast tumors that are identified with genetic testing of these tumors.

Ductal Carcinoma and Lobular Cancer

One way to categorize breast cancer is how it looks under the microscope, and most breast cancers are either ductal carcinomas, lobular cancers, or a mixture of the two types. Thus, the cancer is largely defined based on the initial location of where the tumor originated within the breast. Most breast cancers are considered invasive cancers, which means that they have moved beyond the site where the cancerous cells first began in the breast or they have the potential to do so. These cancers have infiltrated the surrounding breast tissue and they may have also penetrated even further afield.

In contrast, ductal carcinoma in situ (DCIS) and lobular cancer in situ (LCIS) are both precancerous conditions that have not yet grown beyond the original site. Doctors have no way to predict exactly which cases of in situ carcinomas will develop into invasive cancers. However, the American Cancer Society reports that women who have lobular carcinoma in situ have up to 11 times greater risk of developing invasive breast cancer.[2] As a result, if your doctor detects this form of cancer, it should be followed up with regular mammograms and other tests as needed.

Ductal Carcinoma

Ductal carcinoma is a type of cancer that originates in the tubes (the ducts) that send the milk to the nipple when a woman breastfeeds a baby. These ducts are present whether you ever have a child or not and whether you breastfeed any children that you may have or not. According to the National Breast Cancer Foundation, an estimated 70 to 80 percent of all breast cancers are invasive ductal carcinomas.[3]

Lobular Carcinoma

Invasive lobular carcinoma refers to a malignant tumor that starts in one of about 20 lobes located in the breast. Each of these lobes comprises smaller units called lobules. These lobes are the places where milk is produced on an as-needed basis by breastfeeding mothers. About 10–15 percent of women with breast cancer have invasive lobular carcinoma.[4] Others have a combination of ductal and lobular carcinoma or they may have IBC.

Similar to DCIS, some women may also develop LCIS, a precancerous condition. Experts report to women that the odds are about 7–11 times higher for developing invasive cancer with LCIS.[5] However, LCIS is difficult to diagnose with mammograms or clinical examinations, because of the way it grows in the breast, making it hard to detect. Also, there could be no lumps found with LCIS. It may be diagnosed, however, if a biopsy is taken of a suspicious abnormality in the breast.

INCIDENCE OF BREAST CANCER AMONG BLACK WOMEN BY STATE, 2012

The National Cancer Institute and the Centers for Disease Control have studied the incidence of breast cancer among black women by state and nationwide. Some states have such a low incidence of black women with breast cancer that their information is not reported, including the states of Alaska, Hawaii, Idaho, Maine, Montana, New Hampshire, North Dakota, South Dakota, Utah, Vermont, and Wyoming. Data are also not available for Nevada.

Among those states that do report the incidence of breast cancer among black women, the highest rate in 2012 was found in West Virginia, or 148 cases per 100,000 women, followed by Kentucky and Connecticut. The lowest incidence rates were found in Minnesota (78.7 per 100,000), and the next lowest were in Arizona and Nebraska. See Table 3.1 for further information. The reasons for these state by state differences are unknown at this time.

Table 3.1   Incidence of Breast Cancer by Rate and Number among Black Women in the United States, 2012

State	Rate per 100,000	Average Annual Count
United States	120.0	25,747
West Virginia	148.0	49
Kentucky	140.4	241
Connecticut	136.7	276
Louisiana	134.6	1,014
Wisconsin	131.1	196
South Carolina	130.5	956
Oregon	130.4	43
New Mexico	130.1	26

(Continued)

Table 3.1 (Continued)

State	Rate per 100,000	Average Annual Count
Virginia	127.3	1,121
Michigan	127.2	976
Oklahoma	126.8	179
District of Columbia	126.6	257
Indiana	126.2	370
Kansas	125.1	99
North Carolina	125.0	1,471
Missouri	124.9	459
Georgia	124.3	1,915
Illinois	123.5	1,290
Mississippi	123.1	684
Tennessee	121.5	675
Ohio	121.4	938
Washington	121.2	136
Alabama	121.2	840
Maryland	121.0	1,215
California	120.8	1,636
Texas	119.6	1,825
New Jersey	118.3	862
Pennsylvania	117.9	905
Delaware	115.5	124
Iowa	115.4	38
Colorado	114.5	112
New York	112.3	2,236
Rhode Island	112.1	39
Florida	104.0	1,661
Arkansas	102.0	237
Massachusetts	98.4	259
Nebraska	96.0	34
Arizona	90.9	112
Minnesota	78.8	78

Source: Data derived from http://statecancer profiles.cancer.gov/index.html.

Inflammatory Breast Cancer

IBC is a rarer form of breast cancer than ductal or lobular carcinomas, but unfortunately, it is more common in black women than in women of other races or ethnicities.[6] This is not the first time I have made this statement to you, and it won't be the last time, regrettably. There is also a higher incidence of IBC in some Middle Eastern and African countries. IBC is a very dangerous and rapidly growing form of breast cancer. IBC represents only about 1–5 percent of all forms of breast cancer. According to the National Cancer Institute, when IBC is identified, it is often at least a Stage III type of cancer, but it may also be more advanced than Stage III.[7] (The stages of cancer range from 0 to IV and are discussed further in Chapter Five.)

The appearance of the breast cancer in patients with IBC is that of an inflammation or an infection of the breast (mastitis), affecting most of the breast. At times, women are first treated by their doctors with antibiotics because of diagnostic confusion, only to find out after the antibiotics fail to resolve the condition that it is IBC.

With this form of breast cancer, the symptoms often are different from other forms of breast cancer. For example, with IBC, the skin of the breast is thickened, red, pitted, and irritated. The breast size may noticeably increase. In addition, often there may be no identifiable lump within the breasts. Instead, the breast becomes swollen and inflamed, and it hurts considerably. With IBC, the cancer blocks the lymph vessels, causing a fluid buildup that leads to the inflammation and pain. The lymph nodes under the arm also may be swollen, as also the lymph nodes at the bottom of the neck near the collarbone.

The breast may look as if it is bruised. There may also be a discharge from the nipple, although the woman is not breastfeeding. The breast or the nipple may become itchy and the skin of the overall breast may look dimpled like an orange peel. The breast may become warm to touch. Sometimes the nipples retract or even invert inward.[8] However, you need to know that all of these symptoms may also be indicators of another problem, such as an infection or injury or even another type of breast cancer. It's very important for a woman who has these symptoms to see her physician as soon as possible because IBC is a rapidly growing and dangerous form of breast cancer.

In a study of IBC over the period 1992–2009, researchers Bryan Goldner and colleagues found that the highest incidence of IBC occurred among black women (3 percent), followed by white women (2 percent) and then Asian women (1 percent). [9] Although IBC is often identified as a disease that primarily affects women of childbearing age, in contrast, these researchers found that IBC was more prevalent in older women *or* in black women of any age.

Treatment depends on how advanced the IBC is, and it may include surgery, radiation, and chemotherapy. The standard of care is always to quickly start with a strong chemotherapy first. This will be followed by surgery and radiation therapy. In a small study of 55 patients with IBC, including 25 white and 30 black women who were treated over the period 1995 to 2009, researchers Fundagul Andic and colleagues reported that there was no difference between black and white women in terms of their age, the size of the tumor, treatment adherence (whether they complied with their recommended treatments), and many other factors. However, the three-year survival rate was higher for white women (73 percent) compared to black women (55 percent).[10] The reasons for this disparity were unknown.

Some researchers who have performed studies of IBC have also found a high incidence of triple-negative cancer, a serious and aggressive cancer that is also described in this chapter. For example, according to Jeffrey S. Ross and colleagues in their 2015 article, of 44 cases of IBC with bio-marker information, 39 percent of the cases were women with triple-negative breast cancer.[11] Other genetic alterations have also been identi-fied with IBC.

Genetic Classifications

When your breast tumor is typed genetically after you receive a biopsy (a tissue removal from the tumor located within the breast), it will fall into one of four primary categories. These key types are very important for your doctor to know about because your treatment will depend on the genetic type of your tumor. For example, if you have triple-negative breast cancer, which is a type of cancer that has neither estrogen or progesterone hormonal receptors nor the presence of the human epidermal growth fac-tor 2, also known as the HER2-positive protein, then your treatment will be modified accordingly. You won't receive anti-estrogen (like tamoxifen) therapy to treat triple-negative breast cancer because it wouldn't work since you don't have the hormone receptors to receive this form of treat-ment. It would be like throwing a rubber ball against a wooden door—it won't stick. Instead, with triple-negative breast cancer, you are likely to receive chemotherapy.

The four major different genetic types that you will learn about here are Luminal A, Luminal B, triple negative, and HER2 positive. There are some other subcategories of breast cancer that researchers use, so the total percentages of white and black women with these types described in the following sections don't add up to 100 percent, for my sharper-eyed readers. I am concentrating on the main areas you need to know about.

Testing is also done for the presence or absence of hormone receptors, which is valuable information in planning therapy as well as determining the likely outcome (prognosis) in an individual woman. First, I'll discuss hormone receptors.

Hormone Receptors

Testing determines whether a woman tests positive for estrogen, progesterone, and the human epidermal growth factor receptor (HER2) protein. A woman may be positive or negative for each of these factors. If she is negative in all three, she is said to have triple-negative breast cancer.

Most breast cancers are positive for both estrogen and progesterone, and the significance of this finding is that the woman will be responsive to anti-estrogen treatment. Even if she is only positive for one of the receptors, either estrogen or progesterone, she is considered as a candidate for endocrine therapy. In general, the prognosis is better in a woman who can be treated with anti-estrogen therapy. In contrast, when a woman has triple-negative cancer, she will not respond to anti-estrogen therapy and it would be a waste of time and effort.

If the woman is positive for HER2, then she will be responsive to treatment with medications such as Herceptin, but if she is negative, she would not be responsive. If you could pick your subtypes (which you can't), the best one is estrogen positive, progesterone positive, and HER2 positive.

Some researchers have found that an estrogen-positive (ER+) tumor has an increased survivability compared to other tumors in most stages of breast cancer (with an unexplained exception for Stage III).[12]

Luminal A Breast Cancer

Many women with breast cancer, including black women, are diagnosed with Luminal A breast cancer. Up to about 60 percent of white women with breast cancer have Luminal A breast cancer, and some studies, such as by Carol A. Parise and Vincent Caggiano, have shown that this type of breast cancer is present in about 42 percent of black women with breast cancer. These researchers studied 123,780 cases of breast cancer from the California Cancer Registry, reporting their findings in 2014.[13]

Luminal A cancer is usually readily treatable, and it's also a slow-growing form of breast cancer. This type of tumor *does* include estrogen and progesterone hormone receptors, which means that this type of tumor often responds well to treatment with anti-estrogen therapy, discussed more in the section of this book dedicated to treatment. Luminal A breast cancer does not include HER2 protein, and thus it is said to be HER2 negative.

Some researchers say that the recurrence of Luminal A breast cancer is low. In addition, there is generally a high survival rate for many women diagnosed with this type of cancer.[14] Unfortunately, recurrences can occur late in life, and some women have experienced this cancer even 20 years later from the original diagnosis, although this is rare.

Luminal B Breast Cancer

Luminal B breast cancer has a less favorable outcome than with Luminal A cancer, because these cancers are often more aggressive. These tumors usually have an estrogen receptor but may or may not have the progesterone receptor. They are also HER2 positive. (HER2 will be discussed very soon in this chapter.)

Based on the Parise and Caggiano data, there's no significant difference between the incidence of Luminal B breast cancer in black or white women.[15]

The recurrence rate of this type of breast cancer is high. Luminal B breast cancer may be treated with anti-estrogen therapy as well as chemotherapy. Surgery and radiation therapy are also options that are considered.

Triple-Negative Breast Cancer

Sometimes referred to as "basal" breast cancer, or the even more complex name "ER-negative PR-negative HER2/neu-negative breast cancer," this type of cancer is usually called triple-negative breast cancer. Triple-negative breast cancer represents only about 11 percent of the breast cancers in white women, but it is found in a much higher percentage, 25 percent, of the cancer found in black women, based on data from Parise and Caggiano;[16] high percentages of this form of cancer in black women were also found by Stead et al.[17] and other researchers.[18] For example, in one national study of nearly 39,000 people nationwide with triple-negative breast cancer, when the races and ethnicities of the affected individuals were identified, the highest rates were African Americans (24 percent) and the lowest were Filipinos (9 percent). The rate for whites was 11 percent. Clearly, triple-negative breast cancer is a major problem among black women with breast cancer.[19]

"Triple-negative breast cancer" sounds like it must be three times worse than any other form of breast cancer that exists, which is not necessarily true. But if someone were trying to find a very scary name for a type of breast cancer, could they possibly have found a worse name than "triple negative"? Probably not. The reality is that triple-negative breast cancer is not a *good* type of cancer for any woman to be diagnosed with, but that's not how or why this type of cancer acquired its name.

Instead, triple-negative cancer alludes to a type of tumor that does not have receptors for the female hormones, estrogen and progesterone, and thus it is said it is to be "negative" for these receptors. Because it has no receptors

---

TRIPLE-NEGATIVE BREAST CANCER IN WOMEN IN AFRICA: AN IMPORTANT CLUE?

Some researchers speculate that black women in the United States may have a greater risk for triple-negative cancer than women of other races or ethnicities because of long-past ancestors in West African countries, from where slaves were forcibly taken in chains and shackles to what is now the United States several centuries ago.

For example, in a study of African women with breast cancer living in Ghana, a Western African country, the researchers found a very high rate of triple-negative breast cancer. The researchers studied 223 women, and more than half of them had triple-negative breast cancer. The researchers also noted that triple-negative cancer was the most common subtype of breast cancer that they found despite the women's age, their stage of diagnosis, or the tumor grade of the cancer. They also noted that further research into the pathogenesis (the beginning of the pathology) of triple-negative cancer could provide further information explaining its prevalence among African American women in the United States.[1]

With the recent launch in the United States of the Breast Cancer Genetic Study in African-Ancestry Populations Initiative, even more helpful information of the underlying genetics of breast cancer in black women in the United States should be forthcoming. Such information will definitely lead to better treatments that can be offered to black women with breast cancer.

[1]Edmund M. Der et al., "Triple-Negative Breast Cancer in Ghanaian Women: The Korle Bu Teaching Hospital Experience," *The Breast Journal* (2015): 627–633, doi:10.1111/tbj .12527.

for these hormones, it cannot be treated with anti-estrogen therapy. Triple-negative breast cancer is also negative for the HER2 protein, which is the third factor. This type of breast cancer is treated with chemotherapy.

In 2015, researchers in Britain found that another gene, the *BCL11A* gene, had become hyperactive in the majority of patients with triple-negative breast cancer, although it is not clear if this genetic activity is the cause of this form of cancer.[20] This research finding should, hopefully, help improve screening as well as treatment.

Triple-negative breast cancer is believed to be much more likely to be found in women of childbearing age in the United States than among postmenopausal women. Whenever possible, it's best when this form of cancer is identified and treated in the early stages. Recurrences from triple-negative disease tend to occur early, and if women survive 3–5 years without a recurrence, the chances of having a relapse are generally low.

HER2 Positive

HER2 positive is another genetic stand-alone category of breast cancer. In their joint practice recommendations in 2014, both the American Society of Clinical Oncology and the College of American Pathologists recommend that all individuals with invasive breast cancer or recurrent breast cancer must be tested for HER2 protein.[21] The American Cancer Society also makes this recommendation.[22] If the test is inconclusive, they then recommend that further testing be performed using a different means of testing. The laboratory doing the testing should also be one that has been accredited by the College of American Pathologists. (To find out if a laboratory is accredited, ask it if it has been accredited.) In some cases, a new biopsy is needed so that it can be determined if the tumor is HER2 positive or not.

Testing is important because the patient's HER2 status determines whether some chemotherapy drugs are or are not recommended. It is also true that breast cancers that are HER2 positive may be faster growing and more aggressive tumors, which is very important information for the doctor and the patient.

In individuals with breast cancer who are HER2 positive, the condition is generally categorized as estrogen negative and progesterone negative, but it is HER2 positive. About 8 percent of black women with breast cancer (and 6 percent of white women, so there's not much difference) have this type of breast cancer, which is an over-expression of the HER2 protein because of amplification of the *HER2* gene itself.[23] Individuals with this type of breast cancer are generally treated with chemotherapy in addition to drugs that specifically target the HER2 protein (such as trastuzumab,

---

A CANCER RISK ASSESSMENT TOOL FOR INVASIVE BREAST CANCER

To determine your risk of developing invasive breast cancer, which is breast cancer that has spread beyond where cancer began in the breast, consider using the Breast Cancer Risk Assessment Tool. This tool takes into account the risks black women face for breast cancer. Developed by the National Cancer Institute and other organizations, you answer simple questions online about your current age, race, age when you had your first period, age when you had your first child, and other questions, and the tool will determine your percentage risk for invasive breast cancer. If you've already had breast cancer, you can still take the test to determine your possible recurrence risk. The tool is offered on the Seattle Cancer Care Alliance website at: https://www.seattlecca.org/

---

also known as Herceptin), although every case is different. See Chapter Five for more information on who should receive genetic testing.

Also, note that patients with IBC may be HER2 positive.

Mutations in the *BRCA1* and *BRCA2* Genes

Researchers have found that some women develop breast cancer because of genetic mutations in the BRCA1 and BRCA2 genes., The BR stands for "breast" and the CA stands for "cancer." There are two main genetic mutations, affecting the BRCA1 and BRCA2 genes, respectively. These genetic mutations are believed to be the most likely suspects that are responsible for causing breast cancer as well as ovarian cancer, and some other cancers.[24]

BRCA1 is a gene on chromosome 17 that normally suppresses the growth of cancer. Thus, the person with this genetic mutation has a greater risk for breast cancer, as well as ovarian cancer and other types of cancer. This genetic mutation is also more frequently found among younger women and is more likely to be associated with cancer that affects both breasts than without the mutation. Multiple members of the same family may be affected by breast or related cancers. A careful and detailed family history is very important. It may also be more prevalent in certain populations, such as Ashkenazi Jews from Eastern Europe.[25] As discussed in Chapter One, younger black women with breast cancer have a higher probability of having this genetic mutation than postmenopausal women.[26]

With regard to *BRCA2*, this is a gene mutation on chromosome 13, also where the gene normally stops cancer in its tracks. The woman with the genetic *BRCA2* mutation has an elevated risk for breast cancer and ovarian cancer.[27] Some studies have found an elevated risk for these genetic mutations among black women, as will be discussed later.

Genetic Testing

Genetic testing can reveal the presence of these mutated breast cancer genes. The treatment of the individual may depend on whether she has these genetic mutations or not. For example, a lumpectomy is likely *not* the best treatment for women with this genetic mutation because tumors spawned by the *BRCA1* or *BRCA2* genetic mutations are particularly aggressive, and consequently, they are likely to eventually spread to the entire breast. Moreover, these mutations put the woman at risk of developing another new cancer in the breast that is unrelated to the first one.

Precautionary Mastectomies

Some women with *BRCA1* or *BRCA2* genetic mutations have had their breasts removed before cancer has ever developed, most notably actress Angelina Jolie. She is not a black woman, but she is a celebrity whom readers may have heard about. According to Jolie, she had inherited an 87 percent chance of developing breast cancer, and this is why she had a double mastectomy.[28] Although it is possible that cancer might never develop, such women have feared the aggressiveness of the cancer if it ever did develop, and consequently, they made this controversial choice to preempt cancer altogether by eliminating the site where it could develop— the breast.

Notes

1. Lesley A. Stead et al., "Triple-Negative Breast Cancers Are Increased in Black Women Regardless of Age or Body Mass Index," *Breast Cancer Research* 11, no. 2 (2009), http:breast-cancer-research.com/content/11/1/R18 (accessed May 10, 2016); P. Boyle, "Triple-Negative Breast Cancer: Epidemiological Considerations and Recommendations," *Annals of Oncology* 23, Supp. 6 (2012): v7–v12; Bryan Goldner et al., "Incidence of Inflammatory Breast Cancer in Women, 1992–2009,

United States," *Annals of Surgical Oncology* 21, no. 4 (April 2014): 1267–1270; Eric C. Dietze et al., "Triple-Negative Breast Cancer in African-American women: Disparities Versus Biology," *Nature Reviews Cancer* (February 12, 2015), doi:10:1038/nrc3896; Magdalena L. Plasilova et al., "Features of Triple-Negative Breast Cancer: Analysis of 38,813 Cases from the National Cancer Database," *Medicine*, July 27, 2016, https://www.ncbi.nlm.nih.gov/pmc/articles/PMC5008562/ (accessed November 29, 2016).

2. American Cancer Society, *Breast Cancer*, Atlanta, GA, May 4, 2016, http://www.cancer.org/acs/groups/cid/documents/webcontent/003090-pdf.pdf (accessed September 10, 2016).

3. National Breast Cancer Foundation, "What Is Breast Cancer?" Undated, http://www.nationalbreastcancer.org/invasive-ductal-carcinoma (accessed September 23, 2016).

4. Johns Hopkins Breast Center, "Invasive Lobular Carcinoma," Undated, http://www.hopkinsmedicine.org/breast_center/breast_cancers_other_condi tions/invasive_lobular_carcinoma.html (accessed September 23, 2016).

5. American Cancer Society, "Lobular Carcinoma in Situ (LCIS)," April 21, 2016, http://www.cancer.org/healthy/findcancerearly/womenshealth/non-cancer ousbreastconditions/non-cancerous-breast-conditions-lobular-carcinoma-in-situ (accessed September 24, 2016).

6. Bryan Goldner et al., "Incidence of Inflammatory Breast Cancer in Women, 1992–2009, United States," *Annals of Surgical Oncology* 21, no. 4 (April 2014): 1267–1270.

7. National Cancer Institute, "Inflammatory Breast Cancer," January 6, 2016, https://www.cancer.gov/types/breast/ibc-fact-sheet (accessed September 23, 2016).

8. Ibid.

9. Bryan Goldner et al., "Incidence of Inflammatory Breast Cancer in Women, 1992–2009, United States," *Annals of Surgical Oncology* 21, no. 4 (April 2014): 1267–1270.

10. Fundagul Andic et al., "Treatment Adherence and Outcome in Women with Inflammatory Breast Cancer: Does Race Matter?" *Cancer* (December 15, 2011): 5485–5492.

11. Jeffrey S. Ross et al., "Comprehensive Genomic Profiling of Inflammatory Breast Cancer Cases Reveals a High Frequency of Clinically Relevant Genomic alternations," *Breast Cancer Research Treatment* 154, no. 1 (November 2015): 158–162.

12. Carol A. Parise and Vincent Caggiano, "Breast Cancer Survival Defined by the ER/PR/HER2 Subtypes and a Surrogate Classification according to Tumor Grade and Immunohistochemical Biomarkers," *Journal of Cancer Epidemiology* (2014), https://www.hindawi.com/journals/jce/2014/469251/ (accessed April 22, 2016).

13. Ibid.

14. American Cancer Society, *Breast Cancer*, Atlanta, GA, May 4, 2016, http://www.cancer.org/acs/groups/cid/documents/webcontent/003090-pdf.pdf (accessed September 10, 2016).

15. Carol A. Parise and Vincent Caggiano, "Breast Cancer Survival Defined by the ER/PR/HER2 Subtypes and a Surrogate Classification according to Tumor Grade and Immunohistochemical Biomarkers," *Journal of Cancer Epidemiology* (2014), https://www.hindawi.com/journals/jce/2014/469251/ (accessed April 22, 2016).

16. Ibid.

17. Lesley A. Stead et al., "Triple-Negative Breast Cancers Are Increased in Black Women Regardless of Age or Body Mass Index," *Breast Cancer Research* 11, no. 2 (2009), http:breast-cancer-research.com/content/11/1/R18 (accessed May 10, 2016).

18. H. M. Sineshaw et al., "Association of Race/Ethnicity, Socioeconomic Status, and Breast Cancer Subtypes in the National Cancer Data Base (2010–2011)," *Breast Cancer Research and Treatment* 145, no. 3 (2014): 753–763.

P. Boyle, "Triple-Negative Breast Cancer: Epidemiological Considerations and Recommendations," *Annals of Oncology* 23, Supp. 6 (2012): v7–v12.

19. Magdilena L. Plasilova et al., "Features of Triple-Negative Breast Cancer: Analysis of 38,313 Cases from the National Cancer Database," Observational Study presented at the Society of Surgical Oncology, March 26 to 29, 2015, Houston,TX,https://www.ncbi.nlm.nih.gov/pmc/articles/PMC5008562/pdf/medi-95-e4614.pdf (accessed September 16, 2016).

20. Sarah Knapton, "Breast Cancer Breakthrough as Cambridge University Finds Gene behind Killer Disease," *United Kingdom Telegraph*, http://www.tele graph.co.uk/news/science/science-news/11336050/Breast-cancer-breakthrough-as-Cambridge-University-finds-gene-behind-killer-disease.html (accessed March 16, 2016).

21. Antonio Wolff et al., "Recommendation for Human Epidermal Growth Factor Receptor 2 Testing in Breast Cancer: American Society of Clinical Oncology/College of American Pathologists Clinical Practice Update," *Journal of Clinical Oncology* 31, no. 31 (November 1, 2013): 3997–4013, http://jco.ascopubs.org/content/31/31/3997.full (accessed September 23, 2016).

22. American Cancer Society, *Breast Cancer*, Atlanta, GA, May 4, 2016, http://www.cancer.org/acs/groups/cid/documents/webcontent/003090-pdf.pdf (accessed September 10, 2016).

23. Carol A Parise and Vincent Caggiano, "Breast Cancer Survival Defined by the ER/PR/HER2 Subtypes and a Surrogate Classification according to Tumor Grade and Immunohistochemical Biomarkers," *Journal of Cancer Epidemiology* (2014), https://www.hindawi.com/journals/jce/2014/469251/ (accessed April 22, 2016).

24. Ibid.

25. American Cancer Society, *Breast Cancer*, Atlanta, GA, May 4, 2016, http://www.cancer.org/acs/groups/cid/documents/webcontent/003090-pdf.pdf (accessed September 10, 2016).

26. T. Pal et al., "A High Frequency of BRCA Mutations in Young Black Women with Breast Cancer Residing in Florida," *Cancer* 121, no. 23 (December 2015): 4173–4180.

27. National Cancer Institute, *NCI Dictionary of Cancer Terms*, http://www.cancer.gov/publications/dictionaries/cancer-terms (accessed August 8, 2016).

28. Angelina Jolie, "My Medical Choice," *New York Times*, May 14, 2013, http://www.nytimes.com/2013/05/14/opinion/my-medical-choice.html?_r=0 (accessed August 14, 2016).

PART 2

Understanding Cancer Test Results

Part Two includes important chapters on breast cancer health screens such as the mammogram. This part also includes information on understanding your test results from these tests and tests like the biopsy, as well as understanding how cancer is staged according to whether it is present only locally or has spread and whether the cancer is present in lymph nodes, and other key factors.

CHAPTER FOUR

Breast Cancer Health Screens

There are three basic ways that you first may discover that you might have breast cancer. One way is by doing a self-examination of your own breast and discovering a lump, and I'll talk about how to perform breast self-examination in this chapter. The second way is for your doctor (often your gynecologist) to perform a clinical examination of your breast, and during this examination, she may find a lump or a possible problem area that you missed during your own self-examination. The final way to detect breast cancer is to obtain a mammogram, which is a specialized X-ray screening of the breast. In the past, mammograms were performed using regular films, but today most mammograms are digital, which means that the information is sent directly to a computer to further assist the radiologist in making a more accurate diagnosis. The mammogram is a very important imaging test for all women, but especially for black women because of the higher risk for aggressive and life-threatening breast cancers that occur among black women, issues already discussed earlier in this book.

This chapter also covers possible symptoms of breast cancer, although it's important to remember that, when you have breast cancer, you may have symptoms and you also may have no symptoms whatsoever. That's why you need to be screened for breast cancer on a regular basis, including with a mammogram.

If breast cancer is suspected based on the mammogram results, then other tests are often ordered. For example, the doctor often will want you to have a diagnostic mammogram, which is a more detailed screening test than what is provided with a regular screening mammogram. She may also order an ultrasound of the breast, which can offer your doctor further details about the tumor, and/or may order a magnetic resonance imaging (MRI) scan of the breast. The MRI uses radio waves, a magnet, and a computer to take pictures of the inside of your breast. The MRI may also be used in women who are known to be carriers of the *BRCA1* or *BRCA2* genetic mutations, to detect any harmful breast changes that they may have. In addition, a diagnostic mammogram may be prescribed for women with a family or personal past history of breast cancer, even if the screening mammogram is negative.

Of course if your physician thinks that you may have breast cancer, the doctor will probably order some blood tests, since most doctors are known for testing blood to detect possible problems, and the presence of cancer is a major problem. Some blood tests are markers for the presence of cancer, and are called tumor markers. Having said that, however, I would also like to point out that the majority of doctors do not agree on the importance of cancer markers in the blood as a means for the diagnosis of breast cancer.

If a tumor is identified by the mammogram or by any other tests that you are given, then the doctor will order a biopsy to confirm that cancer is present. A biopsy is the removal of tissue from the suspected tumor, followed by the analysis of this tissue by a medical specialist known as a pathologist. It is the only way a definite diagnosis of breast cancer can be made or ruled out. The biopsy and the different ways that this procedure may be performed are discussed further in Chapter Five.

Possible Signs and Symptoms of Breast Cancer

Some women have signs and symptoms of breast cancer, while others have no early warning signs at all and they also feel fine. Note that the signs and symptoms of inflammatory breast cancer, discussed in Chapter Three, differ from other forms of breast cancer.

Also, and this is important to keep in mind, do not make the common mistake of thinking that if the mammogram detects a tumor, then it's already too late. Not true! Some women forego having a mammogram because they don't want to know if they have cancer. Big mistake! In fact, the screening mammogram is intended for exactly the opposite, and that is to detect the cancer at its earliest stages when the cure rate can be high, at times, close to 100 percent.

According to the Centers for Disease Control and Prevention,[1] the symptoms or signs of breast cancer are as follows:

RADIATION FEARS

Some women worry about the radiation dose that they could receive from a mammogram. But the radiation exposure emanating from a mammogram is considered minimal by most doctors, and the opportunity to detect cancer is regarded as well worth the miniscule radiation risk. Also note that this radiation level is nowhere as high as the radiation levels that are received when radiation is used as a treatment to destroy breast cancer or other forms of cancer. According to Robert Peter Gale and Eric Lax in their book *Radiation: What It Is, What You Need to Know*, mammograms prevent 15–20 percent of breast cancer deaths.[1]

[1]Robert Peter Gale and Eric Lax, *Radiation: What It Is, What You Need to Know* (New York: Vintage Books, 2013).

- A lump in or nearby the breast
- A lump underneath the arm (axilla)
- A change in the shape or size of the breast
- Thickened or firm tissue in or near the breast or underarm area
- A discharge from the breast that is not milk. It may be blood or another type of fluid.
- Nipple changes, such as an inverted nipple
- Pain anywhere in the breast, although pain is not typical of most breast cancers

If you have any of the above-mentioned symptoms, be sure to see your physician. You may have another problem altogether, but if your symptoms could possibly indicate breast cancer, it's best to know as soon as possible.

Self-Examination Is Good—But Not Enough

You can—and I think that you should—check your own breasts for a possibly cancerous tumor by feeling throughout the breasts for a possible lump in a process known as a breast self-examination. It should be noted that there some organizations, such as the American Cancer Society, that currently advise against both the breast self-examination that a woman performs on herself and the clinical examination that a physician performs. It says that there is no evidence that either type of examination, whether by the patient or by the doctor, is useful in detecting cancer.[2] The U.S. Preventive Task Force has also taken this position.[3] The American Cancer Society is a wonderful organization, and I've volunteered for it on many occasions. But I have a differing opinion from its. My attitude is that an extra measure of caution without cost and with very minimal effort can't be a bad thing, so I offer some very basic guidelines on how to perform the breast self-examination in this chapter. My attitude is that you can do the self-examination *and* get the mammogram, which is why I discuss some basics on performing this exam.

Most women who do self-examinations check their breasts once a month. Remember, even if you do find a lump, it doesn't necessarily mean that you have breast cancer. That is especially true in younger menstruating women who may even feel a painful lump appearing all of a sudden. It could be a minor problem that your doctor will tell you not to worry about. (But don't ever listen to your doctor if she tells you that you can't possibly have breast cancer because of your younger age! Yes, you can!) If you find something during your self-examination, then you need to see the doctor first and also request a mammogram, to really know if the lump (or another mysterious finding) is not cancerous. If you do find a lump in your breast, it could be a cyst or you could have fibrocystic breasts that are naturally lumpy. However, always tell your doctor if you find something, anything, so that you can have breast cancer ruled out.

Note that some breast lumps that may be worrisome are so small that no one, not even your doctor, could feel them in a clinical breast examination. That's yet another reason why you also need a mammogram to check for breast cancer.

How to Perform Self-Examination of Your Breasts

The breast self-examination can be performed in front of a mirror and while standing up, or in the shower, or you can do the exam while you are lying down. If you are still menstruating, experts say that the best time to check your breasts is three to five days after your period starts. So if your period starts on Monday, then check the breasts sometime between Thursday and Saturday. If you are menopausal, then you should check your breasts at the same time each month for a good basis of comparison.[4]

Many women prefer the lying down method of breast self-examination. It's performed in this basic manner.[5]

1. Lie down on your back, with a pillow underneath your right shoulder. Place your right hand behind your head.

2. Using the middle fingers of your left hand, employ light, medium, or deeper pressures, and starting at the armpit area, make small circles around the tissue of the entire right breast, checking for lumps in the armpits or the breasts.

3. Switch to putting your left hand behind your head and use your right hand to check for breast lumps or lumps in the left breast.

4. Carefully squeeze the nipple to check for any discharges.

5. Whether or not you discover any lumps, make sure you schedule a mammogram as your gynecologist recommends.

Talking to Your Daughters about Breast Self-Examinations

I think that breast self-examination is a really good idea, and I also think that we should teach our teenage and young adult daughters how to perform their own breast self-examinations. You don't have to show

---

IF YOU'RE BLACK AND UNDER 40, YOU'RE NOT "TOO YOUNG" FOR BREAST CANCER

In her chapter on breast cancer in *African American Women's Life Issues Today*, researcher and author Patricia K. Bradley says breast cancer isn't just a disease for older women, although some doctors may think so. Bradley says, "In various focus groups that I have conducted with African American breast cancer survivors, I have heard stories being relayed from women under 40 who were told by a doctor not to worry about a symptom (such as a lump or thickening) in their breast because they were 'too young to have breast cancer.'"[1] This is distressing information because the earlier that breast cancer is diagnosed, the earlier it can be treated. It's also distressing because it's clear that not only black women who need educating about breast cancer. Sometimes it's their doctors too.

If you know a black woman who's worried about a lump in her breast but her doctor refuses to order a mammogram, one idea is to tell her to show the doctor this book. Another idea is to advise her to find another doctor.

[1]Patricia K. Bradley, "African American Women and Breast Cancer Issues," in *African American Women's Life Issues Today: Vital Health and Social Matters*, Catherine Fisher Collins, ed. (Santa Barbara, CA: Praeger, 2013), 66.

them directly, although that's probably the best way. You can also tell them how to do the breast check. Your daughter will probably be embarrassed and tell you to stop talking about this now, Mom! But she may thank you someday if—God forbid—she finds a lump in her breast.

The Clinical Breast Examination

A clinical breast examination is a check of your breasts that your doctor does for cancer. She will physically examine the breasts, nipples, and the underarm areas to detect any changes to the breasts. Often, this examination is done by a gynecologist or a family practice doctor during the annual physical examination check. The clinical examination is usually quick (although perhaps not quick enough for many women!), and it's also an important part of good healthcare. However, keep in mind that your doctor doesn't have superhero X-ray vision to check the interior of your breasts for cancer. That is why you will still need the mammogram. Do you get the impression that I am very pro-mammogram? Then you are right!

The Screening Mammogram

With the screening mammogram, which is the imaging examination that most women receive when cancer is not suspected, you will get undressed from the waist up and put on a hospital gown that ties in the front to expose your breasts. The technician will position you in front of the machine to obtain the best pictures and will then place your breast (one at a time) between two special plates. The test often is somewhat uncomfortable, but it only takes a few minutes. As mentioned elsewhere, be sure to tell the technician if you have had breast implants so that the test can be adjusted as needed. Sometimes implants can block the view to the breast and may prevent cancer from being spotted. And no, the technician can't automatically tell if you have had breast implants, although she might guess if you are smaller person who has chosen implants that are size gy-normous.

Other Tests Your Doctor May Order

If you are at risk for breast cancer based on the findings of the annual mammogram or because of major risk factors you may have such as having other family members who had breast cancer, then your doctor

---

WHAT IF WHITE WOMEN GOT BREAST CANCER YOUNGER AND DIED MORE THAN BLACK WOMEN?

In 2016, the U.S. Preventive Services Task Force recommended in the *Annals of Internal Medicine* that women be screened for breast cancer every two years, starting at age 50. Under this new guideline, women aged 40–49 years would decide for themselves if they should have a mammogram because of familial risk factors or other reasons.[1] In 2016, the American Cancer Society recommended that mammogram screening start at age 45. Other groups have different recommendations for when mammograms should start, and many doctors, particularly gynecologists, are sticking to the "old" standard of starting mammograms at age 40.

But what if the situation facing white and black women today were reversed? What if it were true that white women with breast cancer died at a higher rate than black women? And what if it were also true that white women developed dangerous types of breast cancer at younger ages than black women? Do you think that news would be ignored by white women nationwide?

I don't. I think they would take their pink ribbons and march on Washington, D.C. I think they would burn up Facebook and other social media with their comments, and they would also call up every member of Congress and the Senate. I think they would have a major coordinated hissy fit until that "guideline" was dropped down to age 40 or even lower.

And that would not be a bad thing if white women acted in that way. I think black women should think about whether they are getting a fair deal from these mammogram guidelines because I don't think that they are.

[1] Albert L. Siu, on behalf of the U.S. Preventive Services Task Force, "Screening for Breast Cancer: U.S. Preventive Services Task Force Recommendation Statement," *Annals of Internal Medicine* 164, no. 4 (February 16, 2016): 279–296, http://annals.org/article.aspx?articleid=2480757 (accessed August 26, 2016).

---

may order a diagnostic mammogram. Other tests may also be used for screening if breast cancer is suspected, such as the ultrasound or the MRI scan of the breast. A bone scan and a computerized tomography (CT) scan may also be ordered if there is suspicion of a cancer spread beyond the breast and the lymph nodes. Radiological equipment may also be used in performing the biopsy, such as an ultrasound. The biopsy is the removal of tissue from a possible tumor for the purpose of analysis to see if it is cancer.

The Diagnostic Mammogram

If the screening mammogram indicates that cancer may be present, or if you have had breast cancer before, the doctor may order a diagnostic mammogram. This test provides more X-rays of the breast than are found with the screening mammogram. Women who have had breast implants may need a diagnostic mammogram instead of screening mammogram, but that decision is up to the radiologist.

The Ultrasound for Breast Cancer

If a lump has been identified by you and/or your doctor, an ultrasound of the breast may be used to determine if the lump is simply fluid-filled or solid. If it is fluid-filled, then it may be a cyst rather than a tumor. Cysts are not cancerous.

The MRI

The MRI of the breast may help in the diagnosis of abnormalities in the breast if such findings are not resolved by mammogram. MRI uses magnetic radio waves to make a picture of the breast and help detect abnormalities. The MRI is not a substitute for a screening mammogram. This test may be used in women with family members who have had breast cancer. The MRI may also be recommended if you know that you have an increased risk for breast cancer because you carry the *BRCA1* or

---

DO'S AND DON'TS BEFORE A MAMMOGRAM

Do *not* use any deodorant or baby powder on the day of your mammogram. This could affect your results.

Do tell the technician if you have breast implants because this affects how the procedure is done.

Do share any concerns that you may have with the technician.

Do relax! It'll be over soon. Until next year.

BRCA2 genetic mutations or you have a family history of breast cancer in your grandmother, mother, sister, aunts, or female cousins. The MRI can also be done to reveal any abnormal findings in the chest or abdomen. However, for the latter purpose, it is customary to use a CT scan, which is also simpler and less cumbersome than the MRI. Sometimes contrast material is administered before the MRI is taken to help highlight specific areas.

The CT Scan

The CT scan uses a computer that is linked to an X-ray machine and this device allows the physician to obtain pictures of any part of the body, usually the chest and abdomen, to check for cancer. Often contrast material is given to you orally or by injection to help highlight specific areas of the body with the CT scan. The CT scan is primarily used to check if the breast cancer has spread to the liver or lungs, which are both common sites for breast cancer to spread.

The Bone Scan

A bone scan is a test in which a very small amount of radioactive material is injected into the blood. This material travels through the bloodstream and then it is captured in areas of the bones that have cancer. The bone scan measures the radiation levels in your bones and detects a cancer that has metastasized (spread) to the bones. This type of test may be done if cancer is known or if it is likely to be present, especially in patients with more advanced disease.

The PET Scan

The positronic emission tomography (PET) scan is another radiological test that may be ordered by the doctor but not to make the initial diagnosis. (So don't assume your doctor is doing a bad job if she doesn't order a PET scan for you.) It is used to see if there are areas of cancer spread in someone with known diagnosis of breast cancer in similar way to ordering a CT scan or MRI.

With this test, the patient is injected with a special kind of radioactive sugar, which is then detected by the PET scanner. Your entire body can be scanned with the PET scan. Cancer cells incorporate the radioactive sugar faster than do healthy cells, and thus the PET scan will help to show if cancer has spread to other parts of your body.

MEN CAN GET BREAST CANCER TOO

Although much less commonly found than breast cancer in women, men can also develop breast cancer. According to the National Cancer Institute, about 2,600 men had breast cancer in 2016 and 440 men died of breast cancer in 2016. Men have less than 1 percent of all breast cancers.[1] Men who are the most at risk are those who have experienced high levels of radiation exposure or who have family members with breast cancer. Having high levels of estrogen is another risk factor. Men with breast cancer usually experience breast lumps. The survival rate for all men with breast cancer is about the same as for all women with breast cancer. However, it is unknown whether black men with breast cancer have a worse prognosis than white men with breast cancer.

[1]National Cancer Institute, "General Information about Male Breast Cancer," February 12, 2016, http://www.cancer.gov/types/breast/hp/male-breast-treatment-pdq (accessed August 29, 2016).

If a Mammogram Shows a Possible Problem

If your mammogram comes out abnormal or if the doctor isn't sure if there may be a problem, then you may need to undergo another mammogram, a diagnostic mammogram, and/or an ultrasound so that the radiologist can take another close look at the area in question. The doctor may also remove a small area of breast tissue, so it can be biopsied by the laboratory. The biopsy is covered in Chapter Five. The purpose of a biopsy is to determine whether the breast tissue is benign (noncancerous) or malignant (cancerous).

Blood Test Tumor Markers

In the future, some experts say that "liquid biopsies" may become possible to detect cancer, rather than the currently used and often-painful biopsies involving needles. These future blood tests will check for numerous cancer markers in the bloodstream, and a blood test taken in the regular manner will be all that is needed. Current laboratory tests have not achieved this level of accuracy, and thus when cancer is suspected, the biopsy is still needed to check for the presence of cancer.

For now, some blood tests may be used to detect cancer recurrence and the possible metastasis (spread) of cancer, such as the carcinoembryonic

---

COULD ANNUAL MAMMOGRAMS HELP LEVEL THE PLAYING FIELD AND IMPROVE THE PROGNOSIS FOR BLACK WOMEN WITH BREAST CANCER?

Some researchers have speculated that the poor prognosis for many black women with breast cancer could be improved with annual mammograms. In a study published in 2012 by Paula Grabler and colleagues, the researchers compared regularly screened and irregularly screened women who were black or white and who later developed breast cancer. There were 254 black women in the group with regularly scheduled mammograms and 170 black women with irregular screens. Among white women in the study, there were 726 regularly screened women and 492 who were irregularly screened. A regular screen was a mammogram within two years of the diagnosis for breast cancer.

The researchers found that there were no significant differences between the regularly screened white women or the regularly screened black women. However, among the irregularly screened black women, they were more likely to be diagnosed with estrogen-negative cancers (36 percent) compared to the regularly screened black women (26 percent) as well as to be diagnosed with progesterone-negative breast cancer (46 percent versus 35 percent, respectively). In addition, the irregularly screened black women were more likely to have poorly differentiated cancers (53 percent) versus the regularly screened black women (39 percent). There were also differences between the white women who were screened regularly or not but they were not significant.[1]

The bottom line is that regular screening with a mammogram may improve the disparity and the worse prognosis for black women with breast cancer.

[1]Paula Grabler et al., "Regular Screening Mammography before the Diagnosis of Breast Cancer Reduces Black: White Breast Cancer Differences and Modifies Negative Biological Prognostic Factors," *Breast Cancer Research Treatment* 135 (2012): 549–553.

---

antigen (CEA). The CEA measures the protein level that is normally found in a developing fetus. After birth, these levels drop to very low or zero. When adults have an elevated level of CEA in their blood, this may indicate the presence of cancer. The CEA is considered a tumor marker for breast cancer, as well as for colorectal cancer, kidney cancer, ovarian cancer, and other forms of cancer.[6] Note that some conditions can elevate the blood level of CEA, such as thyroid disease, inflammatory bowel disease, pancreatitis, and hepatitis. In addition, cigarette smoking can increase CEA levels as well.[7]

There are other tumor markers for breast cancer, such as cancer antigen (CA) 15–3, CA 125, and CA 27.29. However, the results of these tests can be skewed by liver disease, pregnancy, ovarian cysts, and kidney disorders.

Tumor marker laboratory information is also sometimes used to identify the possible recurrence of cancer. Note that these laboratory tumor marker tests cannot replace clinical screening by a physician, nor can they replace the use of mammograms or other radiologic scans, such as the CT or the MRI, in helping your doctor detect or confirm the presence of cancer.

Notes

1. Centers for Disease Control and Prevention, "What Are the Symptoms of Breast Cancer?" April 14, 2016, http://www.cdc.gov/cancer/breast/basic_info/symptoms.htm (accessed September 23, 2016).

2. American Cancer Society, *Breast Cancer Prevention and Early Detection*, http://www.cancer.org/acs/groups/cid/documents/webcontent/003165-pdf.pdf (accessed August 26, 2016).

3. Albert L. Siu, on behalf of the U.S. Preventive Services Task Force, "Screening for Breast Cancer: U.S. Preventive Services Task Force Recommendation Statement," *Annals of Internal Medicine* 164, no. 4 (February 16, 2016): 279–296, http://annals.org/article.aspx?articleid=2480757 (accessed August 26, 2016).

4. Debra G. Wechter, "Breast Self-Exam," *MedlinePlus*, February 27, 2016, https//medlineplus.gov/ency/article/001993.htm (accessed August 5, 2016).

5. Ibid.

6. American Association for Clinical Chemistry, "Lab Test Online: CEA," June 6, 2016, https://labtestsonline.org/understanding/analytes/cea/tab/test/ (accessed August 29, 2016).

7. Carolyn Vachani, "Patient Guide to Tumor Markers," Penn Medicine OncoLink, April 28, 2016, https://www.oncolink.org/cancer-treatment/procedures-diagnostic-tests/blood-tests-tumor-diagnostic-tests/patient-guide-to-tumor-markers (accessed August 29, 2016).

CHAPTER FIVE

Understanding Cancer
Test Results

Any woman who receives a negative report on a biopsy—which means that there's no cancer—is a very happy person. In contrast, a positive biopsy indicates that cancer is present, so no joy there. This chapter talks about what a biopsy is, how it is done, and how the doctor decides what to do with the results from the biopsy. In this chapter, I also cover how the information from a positive biopsy may be used to determine how advanced the cancer is, which is information that has a direct bearing on how the cancer should be treated. In addition, I explain the concept of "staging," which is a means that doctors use to determine how advanced the cancer is, using the tumor size, whether the lymph nodes are involved, and also whether the tumor has metastasized or spread to other organs. This is all very important information, so please read this chapter carefully. Then if you have additional questions, write them down to ask your doctor at your next appointment.

The Biopsy

The biopsy is a tissue sample that is taken from the part of the breast where a possible tumor may be present. According to the federal Agency for Healthcare Research and Quality (AHRQ), out of every 100 women with breast cancer who have biopsies, the surgical biopsy will identify at least 98 percent of these breast cancers. The ultrasound or stereotactic-guided biopsies will find 97 to 99 of these breast cancers. Free-hand biopsies (without the use of ultrasound or the computer) will identify about 91 percent of the breast cancers.[1]

The biopsy is sent to a laboratory, where it is analyzed under a microscope by a pathologist, who is a medical specialist trained on how to determine if cancer is present. In most cases when women have a breast biopsy, the results are negative, which means there is no cancer. Biopsies are also redone if surgery is performed for a diagnosed breast cancer, such as a lumpectomy or a mastectomy. The tissues are taken from within the breast and give doctors and pathologists a better idea of how advanced the tumor is and which treatments would fit that tumor.

The time to receive the results of the biopsy varies from a few days to a week or longer.[2] Most women are very anxious to receive their results. If a week has passed and you haven't heard anything, call the doctor's office and find out when the information will be available.

Before the Biopsy

Before having a biopsy, avoid using deodorant on any part of your body and avoid perfume, powder, or lotion. You may also need to stop some medications before your biopsy, such as nonsteroidal anti-inflammatory drugs (NSAIDs like aspirin) or blood thinners (such as Coumadin), which could increase the risk for bleeding or bruising. Ask your doctor if there are any medications you should stop taking before the biopsy and, if so, how many days beforehand you should stop taking them.

You should also ask the doctor if you will need someone to drive you home after the procedure. Find out approximately how many days it will take for the results to be returned to the doctor.

How the Biopsy Is Performed

There are several kinds of biopsies that are used to diagnose or rule out breast cancer, including the fine needle aspiration, the surgical biopsy, the core needle biopsy, or the stereotactic biopsy. Your doctor will tell you which type that she recommends and why she prefers a particular kind of biopsy. If she/he does not provide this information, then ask for it.

Fine Needle Aspiration Biopsy

With the fine needle aspiration biopsy, a very slender needle is attached to a syringe and used to draw out tissue from the area of possible cancer.

This type of biopsy is the least invasive of all choices. The doctor may use a local anesthesia to numb the area from where the sample is to be taken, although this is not always done. This form of biopsy may be used if the lump can be both identified and felt by the doctor. However, sometimes ultrasound is used to help the doctor determine the exact site from which to withdraw the tissue. This type of biopsy procedure only takes a few minutes to perform.

Surgical Biopsy

With the surgical biopsy, the patient is given anesthesia through an intravenous line. This type of biopsy may be performed if there is a high risk of cancer or it is too hard to access the potentially cancerous area with a needle. The intravenously administered anesthesia may make you feel sleepy, and you likely should have someone drive you home after the procedure, for your own safety. If the area to be biopsied can be viewed on a mammogram but cannot be felt by the doctor, then a radiologist can insert a thin wire to mark the area to be biopsied.[3]

In this procedure, the doctor makes a cut of up to 2 inches and removes either part or all of the possibly cancerous tissue. Tissue surrounding the area may also be removed in varying amounts. The removed tissue is sent to the pathologist for analysis. Some women will need pain medication after the surgical biopsy.

Sometimes a surgical biopsy is performed after a core biopsy as when the woman has lobular carcinoma in situ or the pathologist finds a lesion that is high risk although not yet cancerous. The surgical biopsy may also be performed if the first biopsy has a borderline result.

Core Needle Biopsy

With the core needle biopsy, the patient is given a local anesthesia by injection rather than intravenously. The procedure employs a hollow needle that is somewhat larger than the device that is used in the fine needle aspiration procedure; this needle is inserted into the breast, and the doctor removes the tissue that is believed to be possibly cancerous. From about four to eight different samples are taken with this procedure. Ultrasound or X-rays are used to help the doctor find the areas from which to remove the tissue. The doctor may also use magnetic resonance imaging (MRI) equipment to help her guide the needle to the exact spot to biopsy.

The freehand core needle biopsy is a biopsy that is performed without the use of X-ray, MRI, or ultrasound equipment. It is not used often but may be used for lumps that the doctor can easily feel and localize through the skin.

Stereotactic Biopsy

The stereotactic biopsy is another type of core needle biopsy. This is a procedure in which the doctor uses mammograms and a computer to help find the exact area to biopsy and also to help the doctor to analyze the pictures that are taken. This form of biopsy may be used if the mammogram has shown calcifications or a small growth, yet the abnormality cannot be felt or viewed on an ultrasound.[4]

With the stereotactic biopsy, the area to be biopsied is numbed and the physician makes a very small incision. The patient is anesthetized and lies on her stomach. The breast that is to be biopsied will protrude below through an opening on a special kind of table that has been specially designed for this type of biopsy. Sometimes an MRI is used to guide the biopsy. The doctor uses either a needle or a vacuum probe (or sometimes both devices) to remove or suction out the tissue to be biopsied. After taking several samples, the biopsied material is then sent to the lab for analysis. No stitches are required with this procedure.

This type of biopsy is difficult to perform in women with small breasts, so it's likely a different biopsy type will be used in more petite (at least as far as the size of their breasts) women. The procedure is also difficult in very obese women and usually is not done in women whose weight exceeds 300 pounds.[5]

Sometimes with this procedure a very small clip is placed inside the breast as a place holder to show where the tumor is located. It will not prevent or affect future mammograms or cause any harm.

Possible Side Effects of the Biopsy

After the biopsy, some women experience bruising or even infection, although this is not common. Less than 1 percent of women who have had a core needle biopsy will have a more serious complication, like infection, bleeding, or bruising, according to the AHRQ. However, side effects are more common with the surgical biopsy, and about 10 percent may experience severe bruising, while 4 percent may develop an infection.[6]

Some women may also experience pain for a day or so, although this is more likely to occur with the surgical biopsy rather than with the other needle biopsy methods. Contact your doctor if you experience any adverse effects from the biopsy.

What the Biopsy Results Mean

In most cases, the biopsy is negative (no cancer). However, if it is positive, then that means that cancer is present. Sometimes, and maddeningly, a biopsy isn't a "yes, there's cancer" or "no, there's not" kind of result. Instead, sometimes the results are inconclusive, and in such cases, the doctor may decide to wait for a period of time that she feels is reasonable and then do a repeat biopsy later, removing a larger amount of tissue for the pathologist to check. This may feel very aggravating, but "maybe" is always better than "Yes, you have cancer."

Questions to Ask Your Doctor about the Biopsy

It's best to ask your doctor questions about the biopsy before you have it, to alleviate any concerns or anxieties that you may have about the procedure. Here are some questions that you could ask your physician ahead of time:

- What type of biopsy do you recommend and why?
- Will I be awake during the biopsy?
- Will I have any pain from the biopsy?
- What are the possible complications I could have from this biopsy?
- How long will it take to do the biopsy?
- When can I take a shower or bath again after the biopsy?
- How long will it take to get the results from the biopsy?
- Are there any medications that I should stop taking before the biopsy (such as aspirin or other drugs, like blood thinners)? If so, how many days before the biopsy should I stop taking them?
- Will I need someone to drive me home after the biopsy is done?
- Could I have someone in the room with me when I have the biopsy?
- Who will give me the results of my biopsy and explain them to me?

THE LATEST INFORMATION ONLINE: THE PHYSICIAN DATA QUERY

If you want to find the latest information about breast cancer (or any other form of cancer), including diagnosis, treatment, medications, genetics, and many other types of information, check out the Physician Data Query service that is maintained by the federal National Cancer Institute. You can select the information written for patients or that is written for doctors. The website is http://www.cancer.gov/publications/pdq.

Understanding Cancer Staging and Grading

When breast cancer is detected based on the biopsy, the pathologist then studies the tissue sample to determine the type and aggressiveness or grade of the cancer. There are particular patterns to different types of cancers, and based on years of research, pathologists have determined the patterns of cancer that are least and most likely to be aggressive forms of breast cancer. It's also true that breast cancer looks different from lung cancer or other forms of cancer under a microscope.

Considering the Stages

In addition to the grade of the cancer, an evaluation also will be made about whether the cancer has spread to the nearby lymph nodes or has spread beyond the breast to other more distant parts of the body. The pattern and the degree of spread of the cancer cells determine the stage of the disease in a given patient. The stage of the cancer will be determined by the physical examination and the clinical history and by radiology that may include a bone scan and CT scans and certain blood tests. These will be requested by your surgeon or your medical oncologist.

QUESTIONS TO ASK YOUR DOCTOR ABOUT YOUR BREAST CANCER

The National Cancer Institute recommends asking your doctor some basic questions about the cancer, after breast cancer has been diagnosed.[1] (Questions about treatment are included in the chapters on specific treatments, such as surgery, radiation, and other forms of treatment.) Be sure to add any of your own questions to this list:

- Has the cancer spread?
- Do any of my lymph nodes show signs of cancer?
- What is the stage of my cancer?
- Has the cancer spread?
- May I have a copy of the pathology report?
- Would genetic testing be helpful for me and my family?

[1]Agency for Healthcare Research and Quality, Having a Breast Biopsy: A Review of the Research for Women and Their Families, May 2016, https://www.effectivehealthcare.ahrq.gov/ehc/products/543/2234/breast-biopsy-update-160524.pdf (accessed September 12, 2016).

There are five different stages to breast cancer, ranging from Stage 0 to Stage IV. According to the National Cancer Institute,[7] Stage 0 is essentially a precancerous stage, and an example of this stage is ductal or lobular carcinoma in situ.[8] However, even though it is not yet an "invasive" cancer, careful watching and having mammograms on the schedule recommended by a doctor experienced in treating breast cancer are still needed to prevent the cancer from advancing forward to an invasive cancer. Some cancers are aggressive and move quickly and the doctor may recommend surgery. I have also placed staging information in Table 5–1 so that you can quickly glance at it. Stage I breast cancer is considered early-stage breast cancer, while Stage IV is advanced cancer that has spread and is still identifiable as breast cancer cells.

Taking a Look at the Numbers

With Stage IA breast cancer, the tumor is 2 centimeters in size at most, and there has been no cancer spread to the lymph nodes. Two centimeters is about the size of a peanut. However, with Stage IB, the cancer *has* spread to the lymph nodes.[9]

With Stage IIA, the tumor is still 2 centimeters or less in size but the cancer has advanced to the lymph nodes in the underarm area. Confusingly, Stage IIA is also used to denote a tumor of 2–5 centimeters, but in this case, the cancer has *not* spread to the underarm lymph nodes.

With Stage IIB, there are two possibilities. First, the tumor is 2–5 centimeters in size and it has also spread to the underarm (axillary) lymph nodes. (Five centimeters is about the size of a lime.) Alternatively, the tumor is larger than 5 centimeters across but has not spread to the underarm lymph nodes.

With Stage IIIA, there are also four possibilities. The tumor may be no more than 5 centimeters across and it has also spread to underarm lymph nodes or nearby tissue. Another possibility is that the cancer spread to the lymph nodes behind the breastbone. Third, the tumor is greater than 5 centimeters and has spread to the underarm lymph nodes or tissue in the area. Last, cancer may have spread to the lymph nodes that are located behind the breastbone but not to the lymph nodes in the underarm area.

With Stage IIIB breast cancer, the tumor may be of any size, and it has also grown into the wall of the chest or the skin of the breast. The cancer may also have spread to the underarm (axillary) lymph nodes or it could have spread to the lymph nodes behind the breastbone.

Local, Regional, or Distant Breast Cancer

One simple way of describing cancer staging is to say that the cancer is local, regional, or distant. When breast cancer is local, it has remained within the breast and has spread no further. When it is regional, the cancer has spread to the lymph nodes, such as the nodes that are located under the arms or at the base of the neck. If breast cancer is described as distant, this means that the cancer has metastasized to beyond the breast and the underarm and has spread to these areas through either the lymphatic system or the bloodstream.[1]

[1]California Department of Health Services, Cancer Detection and Treatment Branch, *A Woman's Guide to Breast Cancer Treatment,* Sacramento, CA, January 2016.

With Stage IIIC, the tumor may be of any size, and it has spread to the lymph nodes under the arm and behind the breastbone. Alternatively, the cancer has moved to the lymph nodes that lie below or above the collarbone.

Stage IV refers to cancer that has spread to distant areas of the body, also referred to as metastasis. Breast cancer cells in this stage may be also found in the brain, the lungs, the liver, and the bones. This cancer is not curable at this point, but it is treatable, and patients in this stage may wish to join a clinical study where experimental therapies are being used. Therapies are also offered to treat pain.

The TNM Method of Staging Cancer

Although most doctors will give you information on the grouping of breast cancer information that I just described, some physicians may give you the information based on what is called the "TNM" system of staging. With this type of staging, the person's tumor is classified with regard to three items, including the tumor size (the "T" in TNM), the lymph node status (the "N" in TNM), and, last, whether the cancer has metastasized or spread or it has not (the "M"). This system was created by the American Joint Committee on Cancer and the International Union against Cancer, and is used to stage breast cancer and other forms of cancer.[10]

According to the American Cancer Society in its book *Breast Cancer,* with the TNM method of staging, there are seven possibilities of breast tumor findings, ranging from TX, in which the primary cancer site cannot be determined, and up to T4, which is a tumor of any size that is found growing into the skin or the wall of the chest.[11] T0 indicates no evidence of a tumor, which means it is a negative finding. Tis refers to carcinoma in situ, which means the person has ductal carcinoma in situ or lobular carcinoma in situ. With T1 cancer, the tumor is at least 2 centimeters in size. With T2, the tumor is between 2 and 5 centimeters across. With T3, the tumor is greater than 5 centimeters across.

Regarding the lymph node categories in the TNM system, the cancer is staged with a 0, 1, 2, or 3, depending on whether the cancer has spread to the lymph nodes near the breast and also depending on how many lymph nodes are involved. For example, an N0 is used if the lymph nodes cannot be evaluated, as when they were removed in the past. With an N1 rating, the cancer has spread to 1–3 underarm (axillary) lymph nodes or cancer is found in the lymph nodes near the breastbone.

The "M" in TNM refers to metastasis, also known as cancer spread, and the cancer has either not spread, which is 0, or it has spread, which is 1. There are no other choices with the "M" option of the TNM system.

Be sure to ask your doctor for more information on staging cancer, if you have any further questions.

Why Staging Is Important

Staging breast cancer is very important because it determines prognosis and what treatment to receive. For example, if the tumor is Stage 0, surgery may be unnecessary, unless the patient has mutated genes such as *BRCA1* or *BRCA2* or has triple-negative breast cancer. However, if the tumor is more advanced, surgery may be life-saving. Everyone needs to consult with her own doctor to find out the best treatment for the individual because there is great variability in what is best for your own case. If the tumor is not advanced, then chemotherapy may be not needed. However, if the tumor is advanced, then receiving chemotherapy may be a good choice.

Staging also helps doctors determine the patient's five-year probability of surviving. In fact, the woman with breast cancer may actually survive for ten, twenty, or more years, but for purposes of research and for comparison, experts like to look at the five-year survival rate. As a result, with cancer that is either Stage 0 or 1, the five-year survival rate is nearly 100 percent, according to the American Cancer Society. The rates of survival go down as the stage number goes up, and the five-year survival rate for breast cancer that is Stage II is around 93 percent, while the survival rate for Stage III breast cancers of all types is roughly 72 percent. Even with the worst stage, Stage IV and when the cancer has spread to distant organs, some patients live for five years after their diagnosis: about 22 percent.[12]

Table 5.1 Stages of Breast Cancer

Stage of Cancer	Tumor Size	Has Cancer Spread beyond Original Site?
0	Very small	No
IA	No more than 2 cm	No
IB	No more than 2 cm	Yes, cancer cells are found in lymph nodes
IIA	No more than 2 cm	Yes, cancer has spread to underarm lymph nodes
	Tumor is 2–5 cm	No, cancer has not spread to underarm lymph nodes
IIB	2–5 cm	Yes, spread to underarm lymph nodes
	Larger than 5 cm	Not spread to underarm lymph nodes
IIIA	No more than 5 cm	Spread to underarm lymph nodes attached to each other or to tissue nearby
		Spread to lymph nodes behind the breastbones
	Greater than 5 cm	Cancer has spread to underarm lymph nodes that may be attached to each other or nearby tissue
		Cancer has spread to lymph nodes behind the breastbone but not to underarm lymph nodes
IIIB	Tumor of any size	Has grown into the wall of the chest or the skin of the breast. Cancer may have spread to underarm lymph nodes and nodes may be attached to each other or to tissue nearby
IIIC	Tumor of any size	Has spread to lymph nodes behind breastbone and under the arm. Or cancer has spread to lymph nodes above or below the collarbone
IV	Tumor of any size	Tumor has spread to distant points, such as the brain, bones, liver, or lungs

Source: National Cancer Institute. *What You Need to Know about Breast Cancer*. Bethesda, MD: National Institutes of Health, 2012. http://www.cancer.gov/publications/patient-education/wyntk-breast.pdf (accessed August 28, 2016).

Grading of Cancer

Breast cancer is also graded based on certain patterns the pathologist sees in the tissue biopsy. Of course, as a patient with breast cancer, if you had to "grade" your cancer as if it were your student, you'd give it a failing F–. But it's not that kind of grading. Instead, breast cancer is graded as a Grade 1, 2, or 3, and 3 is the worst. Generally, a Grade 1 is a slower-growing cancer, while a 2 is moderately growing and a 3 is more rapidly growing. A grade is another way to evaluate a breast cancer tumor and help your doctor determine the best treatment.

Genetic Testing

If invasive breast cancer is diagnosed, then both the American Society of Clinical Oncology and the College of American Pathologists in their joint guideline recommend that testing for the human epidermal growth factor 2 (HER2) be performed. This testing is recommended whether the

---

WHO SHOULD RECEIVE GENETIC TESTING FOR BREAST CANCER?

Some genetic mutations increase the risk for breast cancer as well as other forms of cancer such as ovarian cancer. The National Cancer Institute says that the following individuals should receive genetic testing for the *BRCA1* or *BRCA2* genetic mutations breast cancer:

- Women who have been diagnosed with breast cancer before age 50
- Women who have been diagnosed with breast cancer in both breasts
- Women who have had both breast and ovarian cancer or who have a biological relative who has been diagnosed with these diseases
- Women who have had multiple breast cancers
- Women with male family members who have had breast cancer
- Women with family members who have tested positive *for BRCA1 or BRCA2* genetic mutations (If you don't know, ask your family members about this!)
- Women with family members of Ashkenazi Jewish/Eastern European ancestry (black women may have such family members)[1]

[1]National Cancer Institute, "BRCA1 and BRCA2: Cancer Risk and Genetic Testing," April 1, 2015, https://www.cancer.gov/about-cancer/causes-prevention/genetics/brca-fact-sheet#q6 (accessed November 29, 2016).

cancer is diagnosed for the first time or it's a recurrent breast cancer. Testing for HER2 will aid your doctors in determining treatment. The tissue taken from the biopsy may be tested for HER2.[13] This test is not used for determining hereditary disease.

Genetic testing may also be performed on certain individuals, to see whether the woman carries the breast cancer 1 (*BRCA1*) or breast cancer 2 (*BRCA2*) genetic mutation. Either mutation increases the risk for developing breast cancer and some other cancers in the patient, especially in the case of first-degree relatives if they also have the gene mutation. (A first-degree relative is a close relative like a parent, sibling, or the person's child.) Women who have any of these characteristics or situations are all considered potential carriers of the mutated *BRCA* gene: women who develop breast cancer at a young age; who have cancer in both breasts; who have a personal history of having had breast cancer; who have first-degree relatives with certain cancers like ovarian cancer; or who have a family history of male breast cancer.

Interestingly, however, some research indicates that black women are less likely to receive such testing than white women, although the underlying reasons for the disparity are unknown. For example, in a study reported in 2016 in the *Journal of Clinical Oncology*, Anne Marie McCarthy and colleagues studied 2,071 white women and 945 black women with breast cancer. They found that black women with breast cancer were significantly less likely to receive screening for BRCA1/2 genetic testing than white women, and this difference was largely based on physician recommendations.[14]

For example, among the black women considered high risk, about half (49 percent) were tested, compared to 75 percent of the white women. The cost of testing may be a factor in physicians' decision, but this is unknown. The researchers concluded, "In summary, racial disparities in *BRCA1/2* testing among women with breast cancer are large and are not fully explained by differences in risk factors for carrying a mutation."[15]

Now that you understand the basics of what breast cancer is in its different forms, the next part of the book talks about what to do about the cancer, whether it's surgery, radiation, hormone therapy, chemotherapy, or even newer forms of treatment.

Notes

1. Agency for Healthcare Research and Quality, *Having a Breast Biopsy: A Review of the Research for Women and Their Families*, May 2016, https://www.effective healthcare.ahrq.gov/ehc/products/543/2234/breast-biopsy-update-160524.pdf (accessed September 12, 2016).

2. Ibid.

3. Ibid.

4. American Cancer Society, *For Women Facing a Breast Biopsy*, Atlanta, GA, August 25, 2016, http://www.cancer.org/acs/groups/cid/documents/webcontent/003176-pdf.pdf (accessed September 24, 2016).

5. Tara M. Breslin and Sandra A. Finestone, "What Patients Need to Know about Breast Biopsies," Medscape, December 28, 2007, http://www.medscape.org/viewarticle/567831 (accessed September 24, 2016).

6. Agency for Healthcare Research and Quality, *Having a Breast Biopsy: A Review of the Research for Women and Their Families*, May 2016, https://www.effectivehealthcare.ahrq.gov/ehc/products/543/2234/breast-biopsy-update-160524.pdf (accessed September 12, 2016).

7. Ibid.

8. National Cancer Institute, *What You Need to Know about Breast Cancer*, Bethesda, MD, 2012, http://www.cancer.gov/publications/patient-education/wyntk-breast.pdf (accessed August 28, 2016).

9. Ibid.

10. National Cancer Institute, *NCI Dictionary of Cancer Terms*, http://www.cancer.gov/publications/dictionaries/cancer-terms (accessed August 8, 2016).

11. American Cancer Society, *Breast Cancer*, Atlanta, GA, May 4, 2016, http://www.cancer.org/acs/groups/cid/documents/webcontent/003090-pdf.pdf (accessed August 14, 2016).

12. Ibid.

13. Antonio C. Wolff et al., "Recommendation for Human Epidermal Growth Factor Receptor 2 Testing in Breast Cancer: American Society of Clinical Oncology/College of American Pathologists Clinical Practice Update," *Journal of Clinical Oncology* 31, no. 31 (November 1, 2013): 3997–4013, http://jco.ascopubs.org/content/31/31/3997.full (accessed September 23, 2016).

14. Anna Marie McCarthy et al., "Health Care Segregation, Physician Recommendation, and Racial Disparities in BRCA1/2 Testing among Women with Breast Cancer," *Journal of Clinical Oncology* 34, no. 22 (August 1, 2016): 2610–2618.

15. Ibid.

PART 3

What You Need to Know about Breast Cancer Treatment

Part Three provides important information on the major methods of treatment for breast cancer, including surgery, radiation therapy, anti-estrogen therapy, chemotherapy, and other newer and emerging options

CHAPTER SIX

Surgery

Nobody likes the idea of losing any major body part—with the possible exception of the appendix, an organ that sometimes causes severe pain, necessitating its removal. In contrast, the breast is linked with both being a woman and sexuality in general. Consequently, the idea of losing the breast is very traumatic for most women. I have known women who said that they would rather die of breast cancer than lose a breast. And they *did* die of breast cancer because they didn't have any surgery.

The first time I had breast cancer, I had breast-conserving surgery because I didn't want to lose a breast, so I understand this feeling. My doctor was okay with the lumpectomy, so I wasn't going against the grain. When the cancer came back years later, I knew I had to have a mastectomy, and so I did have one. I didn't want to die when I knew there was something I could do to live, and I didn't want to leave my son, daughter, and grandchildren behind. I survived the experience and am glad I had the surgery. I had cancer in one breast but I chose a double mastectomy to be on the safe side. I'm glad I made this choice, because tests run after the surgery showed the other breast also was cancerous.

This chapter is about surgery for your breast cancer, including how to prepare yourself before surgery, the different types of surgery, and how to recover afterward. In addition, I talk about breast reconstruction (plastic surgery), which is an option that is available for women who have had a mastectomy. I also discuss common myths about breast cancer surgery, such as the myth that if your body is "opened up" with surgery, then cancer cells will rapidly spread throughout your whole body and kill you. Not true at all. Another myth is that everyone diagnosed with cancer dies from that cancer. The reality is that there are increasing numbers of cancer survivors in the United States today. Per the American Cancer Society, as of 2016, there were more than 2.8 million breast cancer survivors.[1]

Your doctor may recommend surgery to treat your breast cancer, and there may be further choices to make. Should you receive breast-sparing surgery (a lumpectomy, which is a removal of the tumor only) or a mastectomy (removal of the entire breast)? Should you have reconstructive plastic surgery at some point after a mastectomy? You can't make these choices until you know more about them, which is the purpose of this chapter.

Of course, your doctor will give you advice that is specifically tailored to you and your particular case. Your physician will tell you what he recommends and will also inform you of the choices (if there are choices) that you can make. For example, if you have a large and advanced tumor and the doctor thinks it's best to remove the entire breast, it generally would be very unwise for you to have a lumpectomy.

You need to know that surgery for breast cancer, as well as radiation therapy, is considered a local form of therapy. In contrast, other treatments, such as chemotherapy, anti-estrogen therapy, or other drug therapies, are considered systemic treatments because they can affect your entire body. Your doctor may recommend both local and systemic therapy, and will explain her/his rationale to you. If you don't understand something the doctor says, then ask questions. Don't worry about seeming uninformed or even dumb. It's hard for anyone to think straight when they are facing a major life decision like deciding upon therapy for cancer.

Breast-Sparing Surgery (the Lumpectomy)

Your doctor may tell you that you don't need a mastectomy, and that a removal of the part of the breast that contains the tumor is not only sufficient but also unlikely to result in a major cosmetic problem. This procedure is often called breast-sparing surgery, but it may also be called breast-conserving surgery, a partial mastectomy, a lumpectomy, a quadrantectomy, or a segmental mastectomy. There are probably other names that I don't know about or that are yet to be invented. But for now, these terms should suffice for our purposes. Breast-sparing surgery is more likely to be a recommendation for you if you don't have triple-negative breast cancer or inflammatory breast cancer, although the doctor may recommend a breast-sparing surgery in any type of breast cancer, including those two types.

The oncologist looks at how advanced the cancer is, what type of cancer it is, and how fast it's growing, and then makes a treatment recommendation to each individual patient (see Chapter Five). But keep in mind that sometimes the surgeon won't have sufficient information until he opens you up and can see how advanced the cancer is based on the sentinel lymph node biopsy, discussed later in this chapter, as well as other factors.

With breast-sparing surgery, you will have a small scar from the incision, and you may experience a little crease or dimple in the breast as well. Only rarely will women need to consider breast reconstruction surgery after the lumpectomy.

Breast-conserving surgery can usually be performed in an outpatient surgery center rather than in a hospital. You will still need someone to drive you there and bring you home. You can't drive yourself after having a surgical procedure because of the anesthesia you will have received. It'll take about two weeks to recover from this type of surgery, so don't try to rush back to work too soon.

According to the National Cancer Institute, studies have shown that, in general, women who have breast-conserving surgery for breast cancer live as long as women who choose to have total mastectomies.[2] So you are not necessarily making the wrong choice if you decide to opt for the lumpectomy. Of course, if your doctor is strongly recommending a mastectomy, there are always reasons for this recommendation, and you should ask your doctor what those reasons are. If you don't understand the reasons, ask him or her to explain it to you again. If you're still not convinced, get a second opinion from another doctor.

Keep in mind that at least 10 percent of women who have breast-sparing surgery will have a recurrence of breast cancer in the same breast.[3] In such a case, the woman will usually need to have a mastectomy at this later date.

Black Patients ARE More Likely to Have Breast-Sparing Surgery (Lumpectomy) than White Patients

Several studies have demonstrated that black women with breast cancer are more likely to have lumpectomies than comparable white women, although the reasons for this are unknown.

In a large study of 67,000 breast cancer patients, including 48,978 white women and 8,617 black women (the rest were Hispanic or "other"), Tomi Akinyemiju and colleagues reported their findings in *Cancer Epidemiology* in 2016.[1] The researchers found that black patients were significantly less likely to receive mastectomies than white women, and they much more commonly received lumpectomies. This was true whether the black patients had private insurance, Medicaid, or Medicare. The reasons for these findings were unknown. This means we don't know why the black women were more likely to have lumpectomies than the white women. Was it because they insisted on this procedure instead of a mastectomy? Were these women led to this procedure by their physicians? Only further research will shed the needed light on this issue.

In another study in North Carolina on Medicaid patients, reported by Gretchen Kimmick and colleagues in 2006, in the *Journal of Oncology Practice,* the researchers studied 974 patients with breast cancer.[2] Of these patients, 568 were white and 406 were black. The researchers found that the black women were significantly more likely to have breast-conserving surgery than were the white women. Among all the women, significantly predictive factors for having the lumpectomy versus the mastectomy were being younger than age 50, being black, and having a smaller tumor size.

The researchers also found that black women with tumors that were 4 centimeters or larger were more likely to have breast-conserving surgery than white women with this size of tumors: 18 percent of the black women with large tumors had the breast-conserving surgery compared to only 8 percent of the white women. The researchers noted that these racial differences that were found in surgery for large tumors did raise questions about the appropriateness of therapy.[3] Note: In this study, as well, it was unknown *why* the black patients were more likely to have lumpectomies than the white patients. Further research will hopefully reveal the underlying reasons behind these findings.

[1]Tomi Akinyemiju, Swati Sakhuja, and Neomi Vin-Raviv, "Racial and Socio-Economic Disparities in Breast Cancer Hospitalization Outcomes by Insurance Status," *Cancer Epidemiology* 43 (2016): 63–69.

[2]Gretchen Kimmick et al., "Racial Differences in Patterns of Care among Medicaid-Enrolled Patients with Breast Cancer," *Journal of Oncology Practice* 2, no. 5 (September 2006): 205–213.

[3]Ibid.

Should You Get a Second Opinion about Having Surgery?

If you're not sure what type of surgery to have after discussing it with your surgeon, then you should consider a second opinion. The doctor won't be mad at you if you do so, and some health insurance companies require a second opinion. When you seek a second opinion, go with someone who is not in the same practice group as the first surgeon, so you can obtain an independent opinion.

Questions to Ask Yourself about Surgery

The National Cancer Institute recommends that before you decide about your surgery, you ask yourself the following questions:[4]

- What kinds of surgery can I consider? Is breast-sparing surgery an option for me?
- How will I feel after the operation? Will I need to stay in the hospital?
- What are the risks for surgery?
- Where will the scars be? What will they look like?
- If I decide to have plastic surgery to rebuild my breast, how and when can that be done? Can you suggest a plastic surgeon for me to contact?
- Will I need to do special exercises to help regain motion and strength in my arm and shoulder? Will a physical therapist or nurse show me how to do these exercises?

Table 6.1   Comparing Types of Surgeries

	Breast-Conserving Surgery	Total Mastectomy	Total Mastectomy with Reconstructive Surgery
Removal of entire breast?	No	Yes	Yes
Will I have a scar?	Yes, a small one	Yes, a larger one	Yes, a scar from the mastectomy and also one from reconstructive surgery
Will my breast feel the same afterward?	Mostly yes, except for the area where tissue was removed	No	No

(Continued)

Table 6.1   (Continued)

	Breast-Conserving Surgery	Total Mastectomy	Total Mastectomy with Reconstructive Surgery
Will my breast look the same afterward?	Mostly yes, except for the part where tissue was removed	No	You may look different or even better
How long is the recovery period?	About a week to 10 days	About four weeks	About six to eight weeks
Will I need other therapies, like radiation therapy and/or chemotherapy?	Probably yes for radiation therapy and possibly yes for chemotherapy	Possibly yes for both radiation therapy and chemotherapy	Possibly yes for both radiation therapy and chemotherapy
Will I have pain after the surgery?	Some pain	Yes	Yes

The Total Mastectomy

The total mastectomy, sometimes called the "simple mastectomy"—and these two terms sound like complete opposites but they are not—is the removal of the entire breast. A double mastectomy is the removal of both breasts.

With a "simple" mastectomy, along with the breast removal, the doctor usually removes several lymph nodes under the arm. In contrast, with the modified radical mastectomy, the doctor removes the breast, many underarm lymph nodes, and also the lining over your chest muscles. The radical mastectomy is not as commonly performed as in past years, according to the American Cancer Society.[5] If your physician advises you to have a mastectomy, ask him to explain exactly what this involves. And bring your partner or a friend to that meeting, because it may be hard for you to hear this information the first time, as well as remember it later. Many women sort of check out mentally at such high-stress times, and if that happens to you, it's normal, which is why it's good to have a backup person with you. Be sure to ask your helper to listen carefully to the doctor and take notes. Also, ask your doctor for any handout material you can read to explain the recommendations.

During the total mastectomy, the doctor may remove lymph nodes from under the arm to check for cancer. If cancer is present, then you will likely have a modified radical mastectomy.

If you have a mastectomy, you'll have your surgery in a hospital and will likely recover in 2–3 days. Before you leave, the nursing staff and the doctor will instruct you on how to care for the wounded area at home. In addition, the doctor will tell you what to expect. For example, your arm or shoulder may hurt to move it for several days and you may experience some numbness in the chest area.

The Sentinel Lymph Node Biopsy

During surgery, at some point, the surgeon will perform a special biopsy that is known as the sentinel lymph node biopsy or, more simply, the sentinel biopsy. (This procedure can also be performed before surgery if the doctor needs the information to decide whether to perform a radical mastectomy ahead of time.) With this procedure, the doctor injects a radioactive substance and/or blue dye near the tumor, and the injected material visibly moves to the lymph nodes. The surgeon checks for the location where the dye goes first as a first stop, which is the sentinel node, and then removes one or more of these nodes for evaluation by the pathologist. If there is no cancer found in that sentinel node, then other nodes may not need to be removed and more extensive surgery will be unnecessary. If cancer is found in the sentinel node, then more lymph nodes will be removed from a nearby area.[6]

The Day of Surgery

Your doctor will give you advance information on how to prepare for your surgery beforehand. In most cases, you will need to forego eating or drinking anything after midnight so that your risk for nausea and vomiting from anesthesia will be significantly reduced. Your doctor will likely have ordered blood tests to make sure all is well with you. If you take blood-thinning drugs like warfarin (Coumadin) or related medications, you will need to stop taking them before the surgery. Ask the doctor when is the last time you should take such drugs. And if you forget and go ahead and take the blood-thinning medication anyway, tell your doctor and reschedule the surgery! You don't want to have a severe bleeding problem! That is much worse than any embarrassment you may feel for having made a mistake.

Table 6.2   Do's and Don'ts before Surgery

Do This	Don't Do This
Decide that your surgery is a step toward good health.	Ruminate endlessly about everything that possibly could go wrong during surgery.
Find out how much time you need to take off from work and let your boss know.	Tell your boss at the last minute that you have to have surgery and can't come in tomorrow.
Make a plan for who will drive you to the hospital or surgery center.	Assume someone will be available when you need them to drive you.
Fill your prescription for pain medication in case you need it.	Don't fill it. You are tough and pain is natural.

You should have someone drive you to the hospital on the day of surgery. You will be too nervous to drive and you should not leave your car in the parking lot for days. You will not be able to drive yourself home after you recover from the surgery, whatever the procedure.

The staff will ask you when was the last time you had anything to eat and drink and will take your "vitals," such as your blood pressure, pulse, and temperature. The anesthesiologist will go over your current medications and ask you if you have had a bad reaction to anesthesia in any past surgeries you may have had. The nurse (and sometimes the doctor) will set up an intravenous line for the anesthesia you will receive during the surgery.

After Surgery for Breast Cancer: What to Expect

Depending on the type of surgery you have, you may have what some doctors call "discomfort," but which I call by its rightful name: pain. Nobody likes pain, and you don't have to tough it out. There are no extra points awarded for suffering. Narcotic painkillers can take the edge off the pain and make it possible for you to sleep a lot, enabling your body to start the healing process. Don't worry about becoming a drug addict. The narcotics you'll be given in the hospital as well as any prescribed to you for when you go home are carefully controlled. However, if you've had issues with narcotics in the past, tell the doctor and he'll take it into account.

The level of your pain varies with the extent of the procedure (see Table 6–1). If you have breast-conserving surgery, the pain will be less than if you have either a mastectomy or a mastectomy with reconstructive surgery. Hopefully knowing that the cancer is now gone from you will also make you feel much better and will help you to keep your spirits up. The invader is gone!

The nursing staff will show you how to care for your surgery site, and how to manage a drain if one has been used to help your body rid itself of fluid that has amassed subsequent to the surgery. No matter what type of surgery you have had, you need to carefully read the care directions you've been given and follow them to decrease the risk of infection and any other problems that could occur.

BLACK WOMEN HAVE A HIGHER PERCENTAGE OF SURGICAL DELAYS FOR BREAST CANCER THAN WHITE WOMEN

In a study of 304 black women and 330 white women diagnosed with early stage breast cancer, Prethibha George and colleagues reported in 2015 that the black women had a significantly higher risk of delayed surgery after a diagnosis of cancer with a biopsy than the white women.[1] This is very troubling since black women have a higher rate of aggressive tumors. In addition, delayed treatment can lead to a much worse prognosis.

The subjects were drawn from patients in New Jersey who were studied between 2005 and 2010. The researchers found that of the black women who experienced a surgical delay, 20 percent experienced a delay of two months and 7 percent experienced a delay of three months or more to their surgery. In contrast, among the white women, 8 percent experienced a delay of two months and only 1 percent experienced a delay to surgery of three months or more. Thus, the black women had a 2.5 times greater risk of a delay to surgery in more than two months than the white women. Even worse, the black women had almost seven times greater risk of having surgery delayed for three or more months.[2] Note: It's unknown why the surgeries were delayed and further research may provide important and needed answers. We don't know if the women delayed the surgery or they received poor medical treatment. We *need* to know this information so that black women with cancer can receive more timely treatment.

[1] Prethiba George et al., "Diagnosis and Surgical Delays in African American and White Women with Early-Stage Breast Cancer," *Journal of Women's Health* 24, no. 4 (2015): 209–217.
[2] Ibid.

Recovering from Surgery

Your recovery from surgery depends on the type of surgery you have had, and your recovery will be fastest with breast-conserving surgery. Your general health prior to the surgery (other than your breast cancer) may also be a factor after surgery. However, keep in mind that soon after surgery, your doctor may wish you to undergo additional therapy, such as radiation therapy and/or chemotherapy, as well as other therapeutic options for breast cancer. Some of these options can be even more physically and emotionally draining than surgery itself. (See Chapter Seven to read about radiation therapy and Chapter Eight to read about chemotherapy, anti-estrogen therapy, and other treatment options.)

Your surgical recovery may also depend on other factors, such as your general attitude. Please note that I'm not asking you to suddenly become a cheery person right after cancer surgery. That's too much to ask of anyone! But try to see some of the positives. Such as, the surgery is *over*! That was one scary task, and now you've leaped over that challenging hurdle.

General Advice for Recovering from Breast Cancer Surgery

Here's some basic advice for you after surgery:

- Don't be too impatient to resume your normal activities.
- Be sure to rest enough.
- Take pain medications if you need them.
- Give yourself a chance to recover psychologically.
- Use physical therapy as needed.
- Don't assume everyone knows how you feel. (Tell them!)

Don't be Too Impatient to Resume Your Normal Activities

After you have surgery, you may be in a rush to get back to work and to resume your normal activities. Please remember that surgery is a trauma to your body and you need some recovery time. Sure, the trauma was initiated by a surgeon and it was done for your health, but it's still trauma nonetheless. You need time to heal. How much time? It depends on the type of surgery you have had, but your doctor will tell you ahead of time how long you will be out of action. Use that as a guideline. You may recover more quickly than anticipated or it may take you longer. This is not a race. Your body will give you indications if it needs rest, like severe fatigue or escalating pain.

Be Sure to Rest Enough

After surgery, give your body a chance to rest and recuperate. Get plenty of sleep. Don't be angry with yourself or your body because you need some extra "down time." Watch daytime television and those stupid shows about who's the real father of the baby, read books, and sleep.

Take Pain Medications If You Need Them

Some women think they are heroic if they are in severe pain and they don't take pain medications. But when your body is suffering from pain, it's harder to recover and you may feel miserable. If your doctor has prescribed pain medication (and most likely, he has done so), then take the medication at the intervals recommended on the bottle. Don't take more and don't take less.

Here's a secret about pain medications. It's a bad idea to wait until your pain is at its maximal and peak level before you take pain medicine. Instead, if you are suffering from pain from the surgery, and it's noticeable, then take the pain medication at that time, sooner rather than later. (Assuming you are not taking the medicine more frequently than directed.) If you do this, you can avoid those pain peaks altogether. Your body will heal faster.

After a while, you may not feel like you need pain medication anymore, so stop taking them. Also, when you are certain you don't need your pain medications anymore, get rid of them. Do not save them up for some future date when you might need them, which is what many people do. You don't want a visiting teenager or another person to raid your medicine cabinet and think they won the lottery when they discover these drugs that can be abused. If you need pain medicine for some medical problem in the future, you can ask the doctor for the medicine at that time. Some people recommend putting no-longer-needed pain medications in a container with used cat litter or coffee grounds and throwing it out. There are also periodic times when law enforcement collects old pain medications.

Give Yourself a Chance to Recover Psychologically

There's also a psychological process to recovering from surgery for breast cancer. You may find yourself more emotional and weepy than you usually are. You might even worry that somehow your surgery triggered menopause, since you are unusually cranky and sensitive. These feelings are normal.

But if you find yourself thinking extremely sad thoughts that you just can't shake, and they are lasting for weeks or even months, tell your doctor. You may be suffering from depression and you may need to take antidepressants for some period.

Here's one simple thought-blocking exercise. If you find yourself having recurrent negative thoughts, then each time you experience such a thought, say to yourself in your mind, "No!" Imagine it is a very loud No. Each time you experience that distressing thought or a related one, say no in your mind. It may sound crazy, but it often works.

Use Physical Therapy as Needed

After your surgery, you may find yourself very stiff and it may be hard to move your arm or your shoulder. Physical therapy often can help you regain your strength with special exercises that the therapist shows you how to perform.

Don't Assume Everyone Knows How You Feel (Tell Them!)

Although people can observe your body language and behavior, the reality is that other people can't really know how you feel unless you tell them. There is no special thermometer to take your emotional temperature. So do let people know if you want them around or if you just want to be left alone for a few hours. It'll help a lot.

Myths about Breast Cancer Surgery

There are several key myths about surgery for breast cancer that I think are important to address. They are the following:

- Myth: Having surgery makes breast cancer spread.
- Myth: Everyone who gets cancer dies from cancer.
- Myth: If your family has a history of breast cancer, always get a mastectomy.
- Myth: If underarm lymph nodes are removed, your underarm will be swollen for life.
- Myth: You should avoid surgery altogether and go on a special diet.
- Myth: If I have pain in my knees or hips years later, it means cancer has spread to the bones.

Myth: Having Surgery Makes Breast Cancer Spread

This is a myth about breast cancer as well as other forms of cancer, and the myth is that the opening of your body with a surgical incision will somehow make the "air" get to it faster or cause cancer cells to escape rapidly into your bloodstream. Or that something else happens in surgery, and the cancer will then spread like wildfire to your entire body, dooming you to death very soon. This is just not true. Breast cancer doesn't spread through the air or the bloodstream. It spreads via lymph nodes.[7]

Breast cancer surgery doesn't always save lives because sometimes the cancer has already spread when the surgery is performed. But it wasn't the opening of the body with the surgical incision that caused the problem. Instead, it was the extensive growth that occurred well before the surgery ever happened. Also, often breast cancer surgery *does* save lives.

Myth: Everyone Who Gets Cancer Dies from Cancer

Another common myth, and one that stigmatizes people with breast cancer as well as other forms of cancer, is that a cancer diagnosis is equivalent to a death sentence. Of course, some women do die from breast cancer. But millions of others survive breast cancer and other forms of cancer and live long and happy lives. However, this belief is hard to cope with, because the people around you may think that you are doomed and living on "borrowed time."

Some experts say that this belief may extend to the workplace, where employers are hesitant to hire individuals who have recovered from cancer. Because of this common myth, many individuals try to keep their cancer diagnosis a secret from everyone at work. This can be hard to achieve, because you will need to take time off for surgery, and if you also need radiation therapy and chemotherapy, these treatments are debilitating and you may need to take a leave of absence from work.

Myth: If Your Family Has a History of Breast Cancer, Always Get a Mastectomy

Another myth is that if your family has a history of breast cancer, and let's say your mother or your sister (or both) have had breast cancer, then you must default to a mastectomy if you develop breast cancer and not ever consider having breast-conserving surgery (the lumpectomy). Sometimes people go to the extreme of asking to have both breasts removed even when the other breast has no cancer in it! In truth, every person is different, and the cancer that your mother or your sister had may have required a mastectomy in their cases. Or maybe they opted for a mastectomy rather than a lumpectomy. The reality is that you and your doctor should work together to determine what type of surgery is best suited for you.

Myth: If Underarm Lymph Nodes Are Removed, Your Underarm Will Be Swollen for Life

Sometimes when underarm lymph nodes are removed during surgery for breast cancer, you can develop swelling, pain, and numbness. But this is believed to occur in less than 10 percent of all cases. It's a condition called "lymphedema," and it is uncomfortable. However, it's not inevitable, and even if lymphedema does happen to you, often physical therapy can bring you considerable relief.

Myth: You Should Avoid Surgery Altogether and Go on a Special Diet

Sadly, there are people who still believe that you can cure breast cancer (or other forms of cancer) by going on a special diet and consuming lots of vitamins, minerals, and herbal supplements. I don't know if such a diet could be preventive—although it's pretty dubious. But the problem is, once you already have cancer, it's *there* now, and it's not going away no matter how much yogurt or bean sprouts or vitamins or herbal concoctions or anything else you consume. It's Not Going Away. So please don't buy into this type of magical thinking that tells you lies that special diets or special herbs or vitamins can cure an existing cancer. Some women may also opt for other "alternative" therapies with unproven track records. You are risking your own life if you believe such nonsense. The problem with nutritional supplements and alternative medicines is that there is no sufficient scientific evidence to support their use. Please trust your doctor because she will be making recommendations based on evidence-based medicine.

Myth: If I have Pain in My Knees or Hips Years Later, It Means Cancer Has Spread

Another myth after having surgery for breast cancer is that if you develop pain in your knees or your hips at some point in the future, that means the cancer has spread to your bones and is causing you to experience bone pain from metastasized cancer. But what it could mean instead is that you are suffering from arthritis in your hip or bones, and many older individuals get knee replacements and hip replacements because of the severe pain and immobility that is caused by arthritis. If you develop knee pain or hip pain, then ask your doctor what to do. It's likely an aging problem such as arthritis, but it's always best to double-check when you have had cancer in the past.

Having said this, it is always a good idea to inform your doctor when you develop any new symptoms that are causing you much discomfort, and especially if they persist.

Breast Reconstructive Surgery

Breast reconstructive surgery is surgery to replace the missing breast that was removed during the mastectomy. It isn't always done and when it is an option, some patients make this choice while others do not. Breast cancer patients who choose reconstructive surgery may receive one of two basic types of procedures. One option is the breast implant and the other is the tissue flap. The breast implant is the more common procedure because the tissue flap surgery is more complicated to perform, and not every woman is a good candidate for it.

You should ask the plastic surgeon which choice is better for you. You should also check to find out whether your health insurance company has any time limits or deadlines for when the surgery must be completed. You don't want to schedule your surgery for a date that is later than when it would have been covered by your insurance. Think how maddening that would be to find out you were a few months or even a few weeks too late! You may also want to consider a second opinion if you feel unsure of the surgery that has been recommended to you.

In most cases, women who have had a mastectomy will also require radiation therapy and may require chemotherapy as well. Doctors often prefer to delay breast reconstruction until the patient has recovered from all cancer treatments. In general, the sequence of events after a mastectomy are as follows. First is the use of a saline expander, as explained later in the chapter; then chemotherapy and then radiation therapy. When these treatments are completed, a silicon implant may be put in place. (Silicone implants are by far the most commonly used for reconstructive breast surgery.)

With reconstructive surgery for the breast, you won't have the same feeling in the breast as you did before the surgery. You might not have a nipple either, although surgeons can create a realistic-looking nipple, and they can also tattoo an area that looks like the dark part that appears around the nipple, also known as the areola.

Keep in mind that you may need more than one surgery to reconstruct the breast. For example, after a mastectomy, the surgeon who is planning to perform a breast implant procedure at a later date will insert tissue expanders under the chest wall. These are like deflated balloons when they are inserted and they are gradually stretched out over the course of up to six months with increasing amounts of salt water to stretch the skin. Later, the breast implant (if implants were chosen) is used to create the new breast.

After the breast reconstruction surgery, it can take up to two months to completely recover from the surgery, according to the National Cancer Institute.

Breast Implants

The breast implant is filled with either a silicone gel or salt water, but usually silicone is used. In fact, many women who never had breast cancer have breast implants, usually because they want bigger breasts than what nature originally gave them. Keep in mind that breast implants don't come with a lifelong guarantee, and eventually breast implants must be

Table 6.3   Pros and Cons of Breast Reconstructive Surgery

Pros	Cons
The surgeon will try to match the breast sizes.	There may be some differences in the size and shape of the breasts.
You won't have to wear breast inserts and you will look natural afterward.	All surgeries are risky and recovery can be painful.
You will retain or regain your sexual confidence.	Your reconstructed breast won't feel the same as the real breast did. If you have flap surgery, you will also lose feeling at the site from where the fat for the breast was removed.
Mammogram screening can still detect cancer in the remaining breast tissue, although extra films may be needed if silicone was used for the implant versus natural tissue.	If cancer recurs, you will lose the breast implant and won't be able to get another one.

changed out. Implants may grow hard, may break, or could even become infected. They may also shift out of alignment. Thus, the breast implant is not a "One and Done" kind of procedure. Ask your plastic surgeon about how long breast implants last for most of his patients.

Your two breasts should be about the same size, so this is not the time to go with a DD cup size in reconstruction of the cancerous breast if your healthy breast is a B size. The opposite situation may also be true—your healthy breast may be large. In my own case, I had breast reconstruction several years after my lumpectomy. The doctor did a reduction of the other breast and then he did a symmetric change of my lumpectomy breast to match the other one. However, the second time I was diagnosed with breast cancer, I decided against further surgery and did not have breast reconstruction. It's a very personal decision and one that every woman should make for herself.

Tissue Flap Breast Reconstruction

The surgeon can also take fat from another part of your body to reconstruct your new breasts, although this procedure is not as common. This is called tissue flap surgery. The fat may be taken from your abdomen or your back; however, this option is not available for thin women who have insufficient fat to create a new breast. Tissue flap surgery is also a bad idea for women who are either obese or very thin or who have serious health problems besides breast cancer as well as for women who smoke, according to the National Cancer Institute.[8] Be sure to only work with a very experienced plastic surgeon who has done this type of procedure many times in the past, since it's a complex surgery.

Experts say that healing from tissue flap surgery takes longer than the healing that is associated with breast implants. However, a key benefit from this type of surgery is that the new shape of the breast should last for the rest of the woman's life.

As with all forms of surgery, there is a risk for infection. You can also lose muscle strength in the area from where the fat for the new breast was taken.

Expenses of Breast Reconstruction Surgery

There are a variety of costs involved with breast reconstruction surgery, including the fee for the surgical facility or hospital, the surgeon's fee, anesthesia expenses, and prescriptions needed after the surgery. In addition, before the surgery, the doctor will order laboratory tests and

X-rays of the area. Even when health insurance covers breast reconstruction, it may not cover 100 percent of the costs involved. Be sure to check with your health insurance company beforehand to find out what is and what is not covered.

DIFFERENCES IN BREAST RECONSTRUCTION RATES BY RACE

Some studies of black women have shown that they have a lower rate of breast reconstruction than white women. For example, in a study of more than 45,000 women younger than age 65 who had breast cancer, published in *Women's Health Issues* in 2014 by T. P. Shippee and colleagues, the researchers found that white women were significantly more likely than black, Hispanic, or Asian women to have breast reconstruction after mastectomy. In addition, they also found that the women least likely to have breast reconstruction were minority women receiving Medicaid.[1]

However, sometimes this possible bias is not borne out. For example, in another study of women who underwent postmastectomy breast reconstruction and who were eligible for care by the Department of Defense (DoD) Military Healthcare System, researcher Lindsey Enewold and colleagues studied nearly 3,000 white women and 708 black women, reporting their findings in *Cancer* in 2014.[2] The researchers said they found no racial disparities between the white and black women with regard to their rates of breast reconstruction.

Breast reconstruction has become increasingly popular in recent years. The researchers also found that breast reconstruction rates increased significantly over time for both black and white women. For example, in 1998, the rate of breast reconstruction was 27 percent for black women and that rate increased to 40 percent by 2007. For white women, the rate of postmastectomy breast reconstruction was 22 percent in 1998 and increased to 41 percent in 2007.[3]

The researchers speculated that other studies that *do* show racial disparities in rates of breast reconstruction may be caused by unequal access to health care, which was not a problem for the DoD beneficiaries.

[1]T. P. Shippee et al., "Health Insurance Coverage and Racial Disparities in Breast Reconstruction after Mastectomy," *Women's Health Issues* 24, no. 3 (2014): e261–e269.

[2]Lindsey Enewold et al., "Breast Reconstruction after Mastectomy among Department of Dense Beneficiaries by Race," *Cancer* 120, no. 19 (October 1, 2014): 3033–3039.

[3]Ibid.

Have Regular Checkups after Breast Cancer Surgery

To be on the safe side, you should continue to have regular checkups and mammograms even years after surgical treatment for breast cancer. For example, if you have cancer in one breast and surgical treatment to get rid of the cancer, it is (unhappily) possible that you could develop cancer in the other breast too. Also, see your oncologist on the schedule that he or she recommends for you. Be sure to read Chapter Ten on following up after your treatments for breast cancer have been completed.

Notes

1. American Cancer Society, "What Are the Key Statistics about Breast Cancer?" May 4, 2016, http://www.cancer.org/cancer/breastcancer/detailedguide/breast-cancer-key-statistics (accessed August 8, 2016).

2. National Cancer Institute, "Surgery Choices for Women with DCIS or Breast Cancer," January 19, 2015, https://www.cancer.gov/types/breast/surgery-choices (accessed September 24, 2016).

3. Ibid.

4. National Cancer Institute, *What You Need to Know about Breast Cancer*, Bethesda, MD, August 2012, https://www.cancer.gov/publications/patient-education/wyntk-breast.pdf (accessed September 24, 2016).

5. American Cancer Society, *Breast Cancer*, Atlanta, GA, May 4, 2016, http://www.cancer.org/acs/groups/cid/documents/webcontent/003090-pdf.pdf (accessed September 10, 2016).

6. National Cancer Institute, "Sentinel Node Lymph Biopsy," August 11, 2011, https://www.cancer.gov/about-cancer/diagnosis-staging/staging/sentinel-node-biopsy-fact-sheet (accessed September 24, 2016).

7. M. Daher, "Cultural Beliefs and Values in Cancer Patients," *Annals of Oncology* 22, Supp. 3 (2012): iii66–iii69.

8. National Cancer Institute, "Surgery Choices for Women with DCIS or Breast Cancer," January 19, 2015, https://www.cancer.gov/types/breast/surgery-choices (accessed September 24, 2016).

CHAPTER SEVEN

Radiation Therapy

Contrary to popular opinion, you won't glow in the dark after having radiation therapy from an external device nor will you set off the clicking of a Geiger counter that detects radiation, in the unlikely event that someone passed you by with such a device. Radiation is often a good treatment to aid in eradicating breast cancer, which is also why it's also another common treatment for many women. There are different forms of radiation treatment, but the common denominator of them all is that the radiation works to destroy the cancer cells—and may also damage healthy tissues, near the cancerous tumor, although radiation oncologists try to minimize this damage as much as possible.

If your doctor says that you need a mastectomy to treat your breast cancer, the odds are also high that he will also recommend radiation therapy as well as chemotherapy, for a triple-pronged approach to knock out that cancer. In addition, if you have breast-conserving surgery (the lumpectomy), you are very likely to receive radiation therapy to that breast. However, there are some unexplained treatment disparities between black women and white women with breast cancer. For example, according to the American Cancer Society Cancer Action Network, 72 percent of white women receive radiation after breast-conserving surgery, compared to only 61 percent of black women.[1] (No reasons for this disparity are provided.) Other researchers have also found that black women with breast cancer are less likely to receive radiation therapy than white women.[2] It's important to know this when you are a black woman with breast cancer because maybe radiation therapy would be the right treatment for you. If your doctor rules out radiation therapy, you should ask him why. You may also wish to get a second opinion. The doctor may be completely right but it's always good to get the view of another expert when you're in doubt.

Radiation therapy, also sometimes known by doctors as simply radiotherapy, has some side effects, and some of them can cause significant discomfort. Some people may believe that black women are "safer" from radiation damage because of a greater level of skin pigment in the skin. Sadly, this is not true. For example, no matter what your race, radiation treatments may cause your skin in the area of the radiation to become irritated, and researchers have found no racial or ethnic differences in the toxicity of responses among women who have undergone radiation therapy for breast cancer.[3]

Radiation therapy as a treatment against breast cancer uses gamma rays, X-rays, neutrons, protons, or other radiological sources to eradicate cancer cells as well as shrink cancerous tumors. The radiation damages the DNA of the cancer cells and other cells and leads to the killing of those cells. In contrast, when you receive diagnostic dental X-rays or X-rays of other parts of your body (such as a chest X-ray if bronchitis or cracked ribs are suspected), low levels of radiation are used to create a picture of your internal bones or organs. However, for cancer treatment, much higher dosages of radiation are used to kill the cancer cells. You will also need repeated treatments at a schedule determined by your doctor because the radiation doesn't work right away—it takes time to kill the cancer. Radiation therapy is usually administered over several weeks and on a daily basis, except for weekends.

DON'T MISS YOUR RADIATION APPOINTMENTS

Researchers have found that individuals who missed two or more scheduled radiation treatments, even when those treatments are made up later, may have a worse outcome than patients who regularly attend their scheduled radiation sessions. Doctors believe that part of the reason for this worse prognosis is the prolonging of the intervals of the radiation therapy that could allow cancer cells to recover. They also suspect that noncompliance with radiation sessions may indicate that patients are also noncompliant with their other treatments like chemotherapy or they may have unmet mental health needs.[1] Whatever the reasons, whenever possible, faithfully keep to your radiation appointment schedule.

[1]National Cancer Institute, "Missed Radiation Therapy Sessions Increase Risk of Cancer Recurrence," February 26, 2016, https://www.cancer.gov/news-events/cancer-currents-blog/2016/missed-radiation-therapy (accessed September 14, 2016).

There are two major types of radiation therapy, external and internal radiation. Radiation that is administered from outside the body is called external beam radiation therapy or EBRT, and when radioactive material is introduced into the body, it is referred to as brachytherapy. EBRT is the most common type of radiation therapy that is used to treat breast cancer.[4] There are also different categories of EBRT, such as intensity modulated radiation therapy, 3-D conformal radiation therapy, and hypofractionated radiation therapy. They are each very precisely targeted forms of radiation that focus and concentrate the radiation on the cancerous area and leave the healthy parts of your body alone as much as possible. Your doctor will analyze your individual case of breast cancer and decide what the best type of radiation is for you.

Radiation May Be Given before, after, or Even during Surgery

Radiation treatment for breast cancer can be delivered before or after surgery, and occasionally, it is given during surgery. The latter is a newer and controversial approach that is referred to as "intraoperative radiation." With this procedure, a single massive dose of radiation is administered during a lumpectomy after the cancerous tissue is removed. Intraoperative radiation is available only at major medical centers, and physicians disagree on whether it is a better choice than EBRT.[5]

Radiation treatment is usually given separately from chemotherapy or at times within the same time frame as chemotherapy. Your oncologists are responsible for coming up with the best plan for you. A radiation oncologist is a cancer doctor who is an expert in radiation treatment for cancer. In contrast, a medical oncologist is a doctor who concentrates on making a plan for and providing chemotherapy and other drugs such as anti-estrogen agents. Your surgeon is also an oncologist, and may be called a surgical oncologist, although more frequently, she is simply called the "breast surgeon."

Before Treatment

Before your radiation therapy starts, you will meet with a radiation oncologist, who will review your case and talk to you about the type of treatments he recommends and the approximate number of sessions you are likely to need.

With EBRT, once a treatment plan is made and agreed upon with you, the doctor will draw colored dots or even a small tattoo of the area to be irradiated. Be sure that you don't attempt to remove these markings because they will provide an important road map for your doctor, sort of a special body MapQuest for the radiation oncologist. Also, if you find that these marks are starting to fade before all your treatments are completed, then be sure to tell the doctor, who may wish to redo them.

External Beam Radiation Therapy

EBRT is radiation delivered to your body with the use of a large machine that is available in a hospital or a treatment center. The machine, which is often a device called a linear accelerator, delivers photon beams in the form of gamma rays or X-rays streamed to the targeted site. It almost sounds like science fiction, like the "photon torpedoes" from an old *Star Trek* episode—but instead, it's very real.

EBRT treatments are given to you as an outpatient. Women will receive treatment daily for five days a week over a three- to six-week period, with weekends off. However, the treatment regimen is entirely up to your doctor, and you may need treatments for a shorter or a longer period. Some forms of radiation therapy follow a shorter schedule and with more intense radiation given each time. This is also referred to as accelerated breast irradiation, and the time frames vary with the procedure as well as with the radiation oncologist.

The treatments themselves don't last long, and you may find that you wait in the waiting room for your appointment for a longer period than the time you actually spend experiencing the treatment. The actual radiation part of the treatment lasts for no more than 5 minutes, and most of the time during treatment is used in setting you up into the exact right position.

Positioning is extremely important to ensure the radiation is targeted very precisely to the cancerous area on your breast. You must lie very still during your treatments. The radiation therapist will be in another room at these times but will be able to see and hear you and can communicate with you. When you receive EBRT, you will lie down and receive treatment from a large machine that moves around you and never touches you. With breast cancer, the area to be irradiated is the side of the chest where the cancer was found. However, EBRT is also used to treat other forms of cancer, such as cancers of the head or neck and other types of cancers. So, others in the waiting room with you may have breast cancer or they could be receiving their radiation treatment for another type of cancer.

You do not need anyone to accompany you for these daily treatments because no immediate side effects occur during a treatment session. However, you may wish to bring a relative or friend to the very first treatment, to help allay your fears.

RADIATION AFTER LUMPECTOMY REDUCES
BREAST CANCER RECURRENCE RISK

According to the National Cancer Institute, research has demonstrated that radiation therapy after breast-conserving surgery (the lumpectomy) decreases the relative risk of a 10-year recurrence of breast cancer by nearly 50 percent. Radiation treatments may work by destroying microscopic disease that had remained in the breast after surgery. Women who benefit the most are those who have had estrogen receptor–positive tumors.[1]

[1]National Cancer Institute, "Radiation Therapy after Brest-Conserving Surgery Improves Survival," December 2, 2011, https://www.cancer.gov/types/breast/research/radiation-improves-survival (accessed September 15, 2016).

Brachytherapy

With brachytherapy, which is also known as internal radiation therapy, instead of using a large machine to irradiate the breast cancer tumor, radioactive material is used, which destroys the breast cancer from within the body. With this type of radiation therapy, the radiation may be either interstitial or intracavity brachytherapy. In general, brachytherapy is used much less frequently than EBRT for breast cancer, although it has become increasingly used. It is also used more frequently among patients with breast cancer who are 50 years and older. In a study of nearly 46,000 patients with breast cancer treated from 2003 to 2010, Grace L. Smith and colleagues found that the use of brachytherapy increased from less than 1 percent in 2003 to about 5 percent in 2010 among patients with breast cancer who were younger than age 50. For patients 50 and older, the use of brachytherapy increased from 2 percent to 11 percent over the same period.[6]

Interstitial Brachytherapy

Interstitial brachytherapy is radiation contained in tiny pellets that are delivered directly to the tumor location through tiny catheters. If interstitial brachytherapy is used, it may occur daily for about a week, although your doctor will decide what the right schedule is for you. However, this method is used less frequently today than intracavity brachytherapy. In addition, because the pellets *are* radioactive, treatment may be given in a hospital.

Intracavity Brachytherapy

With intracavity brachytherapy, an incision is made and a special device is inserted into the breast through a tiny catheter. Some examples of such devices are the Axxent®, the Contura®, the MammoSite®, and the Savi®. After insertion, the inserted end is expanded so that it will remain in place during treatment. Tiny irradiated pellets are sent to the breast through this catheter and left in place for a short period of time. These treatments are usually performed twice a day for five days, although the schedule is set by the radiation oncologist. When the treatment is completed, the device is then collapsed and taken out.[7]

While the treatment is ongoing, the radiation travels like a heat-seeking missile to the cancer, for the sole purpose of killing the cancer cells. As with all forms of treatment, there are side effects to brachytherapy, such as bruising and redness to the skin, pain, and possible infection to the insertion site.

On the Day of Treatment

Wear comfortable and loose-fitting clothes on your treatment days because you will need to remove your clothes before radiation therapy

---

TAKE GOOD CARE OF YOUR SKIN DURING AND AFTER RADIATION TREATMENTS

According to the National Cancer Institute, it's best to take good care of your skin during radiation treatments.[1] Here are some suggestions:

- Take warm but not hot showers and only shower once a day.
- If you prefer to take baths, you can take two baths per week, for no more than 30 minutes each time.
- Avoid ice packs, heating pads, or bandages on the area of your skin that is being irradiated.
- If your skin really hurts in the area that was irradiated, tell your doctor.
- Use soft cotton bed sheets for your bed during treatment.
- Ask your doctor which skin products are best for you to use during the course of your treatment.

[1]National Cancer Institute, "What to Do about Mild Skin Changes," April 2010, https://www.cancer.gov/publications/patient-education/radiation-side-effect-skin.pdf (accessed August 5, 2016).

and it'll be easier for you if these clothes can be taken off quickly and easily. You will wear a hospital gown during treatment, but your skin may feel irritated afterward and it won't feel good to put on tight-fitting clothes when your treatment is over.

Go to the treatment center and sign in. To combat any nerves, bring a book or crossword puzzle with you or a laptop.

After Treatments

After each treatment, you may experience some side effects, or you may not. Many people do experience at least a few side effects, such as skin burns or itching skin but these happen over the course of weeks rather than immediately after starting treatment. Ask your doctor what side effects should be reported to him.

Common Side Effects of Radiation

After you have had your radiation therapy, your skin may be irritated, itchy, and dry. Do not use any creams or lotions unless you have first asked your doctor or his assistant if it's all right to do so. Your clothes may feel tight, especially your bra, so it's a good idea to wear loose-fitting cotton clothes while your body recovers. You may wish to skip the bra for a few weeks or longer, until the area feels more normal and less irritated.

There are several side effects that may occur subsequent to radiation therapy, and they may include the following:

- Irritated skin and burns
- Breast changes
- Fatigue or exhaustion
- Nausea and vomiting
- Low blood cell counts

Irritated Skin and Skin Changes

It's very common for radiation to cause skin irritation and burns. In my own case, the burns from external beam radiation did hurt me, and after talking to my doctor about it and receiving the go-ahead, I used aloe vera cream to treat the burns. Ask your doctor what you should use to treat

---

QUESTIONS TO ASK YOUR RADIATION ONCOLOGIST

The National Cancer Institute recommends that you ask your radiation oncologist the following questions:[1]

- What is the purpose of radiation in my case? To shrink the tumor? To stop cancer spread? To decrease the risk of cancer coming back?
- What type of radiation therapy should I consider?
- Will treatments affect my lifestyle in any way? If so, in what ways?
- When will treatment start? When will it end? How often will I have treatment?
- Will radiation therapy harm my skin?
- What side effects may I experience, and how long will they last?
- Will radiation treatment change my body's appearance? If so, how?
- Will radiation make me at higher risk for any other health problems? If so, what are they?
- How can I prepare for treatment beforehand?
- What can I do to take care of myself before, during, and after treatments?
- How will my chest look afterward?
- How will I feel during treatment?
- How will we know that the treatment is working?
- Are there any lasting effects to radiation therapy? If so, what are they?
- What is the chance that the cancer in my breast could come back?

[1]American Cancer Society, *A Guide to Radiation Therapy*, Atlanta, GA, June 30, 2015.

---

your skin if it is irritated after radiation treatments. Don't use just any product that you may find in your medicine cabinet—some creams or ointments could make the situation much worse! Like pouring vinegar on cut skin!

Your skin will eventually heal up, although the treated area may remain darker than the rest of your skin, according to the American Cancer Society.[8]

When you take a shower, let the water run over the irradiated part of your chest. Do not scrub that area with soap or even a plain washcloth. Also, avoid using ice or a heating pad on the treated area until the treatment team tells you it is okay to do so.

Breast Changes and Breast Pain

Experts report that external beam therapy sometimes causes the breast to become firmer and also smaller. Breast discomfort or even pain may also become a problem. It may also cause difficulties in women who wish to breastfeed their children later in life.[9] The breast and especially the nipple may become either more or less sensitive subsequent to EBRT.[10]

Fatigue or Exhaustion

The tiredness that you may feel after a treatment with radiation therapy is not the type of fatigue that you are used to, such as the fatigue that occurs after you've done an exercise workout or when you have performed more physical activity than usual. Instead, this is a deep-down fatigue that is more comparable to complete exhaustion. If you feel this way, it's normal and you don't need to worry about it. You'll gradually get your energy back again when your treatments are completed.

Some people become so fatigued that they cannot continue to work, and they need to take medical leave from their jobs. Be sure to verify that your health insurance will continue while you are on medical leave.

According to the National Cancer Institute, fatigue among women with breast cancer is exacerbated by the following factors:

- Working while receiving radiation therapy
- Having children still at home
- Anxiety and/or depression
- Difficulty with sleeping
- Younger age
- Being underweight
- Having advanced cancer or other medical problems[11]

Fatigue may also be caused by anemia, infection, stress, pain, dehydration, inadequate food intake caused by a lack of appetite, and other causes. Tell your doctor if you experience fatigue during radiation treatments or any other cancer treatments that you receive so your physician can determine if it's the "regular" fatigue or something more.

Nausea and Vomiting

In most cases, you will *not* experience nausea and vomiting from radiation therapy to the breast area alone. However, if you have an advanced case of breast cancer and any parts of your digestive system are irradiated, such as your stomach or your liver, then you could experience some nausea and vomiting after the radiation therapy. You may also experience nausea or vomiting if you receive high rates of radiation. Your doctor should warn you ahead of time if this is a possible side effect of your treatment. Better yet, ask the doctor what types of side effects that you might expect, so you'll be ready for them if they happen. Your doctor may prescribe an anti-nausea medication to decrease or end the nausea and vomiting.

Low Blood Cell Counts

Sometimes radiation therapy can affect your white and your red blood cell counts. In my case, the radiation dropped my blood cell count pretty low, and then I started chemotherapy along with the radiation therapy and my white blood cell count dropped so low that with my first chemotherapy treatment I had to get Neupogen® (filgrastim) injections to keep my white blood cell counts up for the next chemotherapy treatment. This is a manmade drug that stimulates white blood cell production. Don't worry, this probably won't happen to you. But it is one key reason why the doctor will want to monitor your blood levels during the course of your treatment by ordering a complete blood count test at periodic intervals.

Your red blood cells are measured by the amount of hemoglobin in your blood, and if this level drops too low, then you are anemic. This may also be the cause if you are experiencing an extreme form of fatigue and shortness of breath upon exertion because these are symptoms of anemia. Your white blood cells are also important for your health because they work to fight off infection. If your white blood cell count is too low, then it is difficult or impossible for your body to tackle even minor infections.[12] Having said that, it should be mentioned that low white cell counts leading to infection in someone receiving radiation therapy would be very unusual.

When it comes to hemoglobin, a blood count of less than 8 is of concern to the doctor. With regard to white blood cells, which are the cells that help you fight off disease, a count of neutrophils (a type of white blood cell) that is less than 1,000 is a sign of a potential problem.[13] Please also be aware that a low neutrophil count can also be seen in black women even without receiving any treatment.

If your blood counts are too low, the doctor may wish to delay radiation treatments until you recover to a more normal level.

BLACK WOMEN WITH BREAST CANCER ARE LESS LIKELY TO RECEIVE RADIATION THERAPY AND HORMONE THERAPY THAN OTHER RACES

- Studies of large populations of women with breast cancer who were on Medicaid in New York and California revealed that African American women were less likely to receive radiation therapy than white women. In this study, reported in 2016, there were more than 80,000 patients in New York and greater than 121,000 patients in California. There were about 59,000 white patients in New York and nearly 11,000 African American patients. In California, there were about 81,000 white patients and about 8,000 African American patients.

- Based on their stages and general recommended treatments, the researchers found that the African American women were significantly less likely to receive radiation, surgery, or hormone therapy, although they were more likely than white patients to receive chemotherapy. The researchers did not know the cause of the disparities that they found but suggested that factors such as accessible health care, geographic variations, hospital/provider characteristics, and patient preferences may have all played roles.[1]

- If black women are less likely to receive radiation therapy or other life-sustaining treatments for breast cancer—and a significant body of research indicates that this is a problem—then it's important to identify the actual factors that lie behind these disparities. Discovering why black patients are treated much differently than other patients with breast cancer is very important in improving their health care, not only for black women with breast cancer but also for all black women.

[1] Michael J. Hassett et al., "Variation in Breast Cancer Care Quality in New York and California Based on Race/Ethnicity and Medicaid Enrollment," *Cancer* 122 (2016): 420–431.

When Radiation Treatments Are Completed

After your radiation therapy treatments are completely over, you will discuss other possible needed treatments with your doctor. The doctor may also wish to order more laboratory tests or she may order imaging tests such as a CT scan, an MRI, or a PET scan. You may need anti-estrogen therapy and/or chemotherapy, as well as other possible treatments discussed in the next chapter.

Myths about Radiation Therapy

As with most medical therapies, there is an array of different myths about radiation therapy. Here are some of the more prominent myths that you may hear, along with the reality of each situation.

- EBRT makes you radioactive and dangerous to others.
- Radiation therapy destroys all your skin.
- Radiation makes you bald.
- Radiation treatments kill the cancer so it can never come back.
- Radiation therapy is painful.

Myth: External Beam Radiation Therapy Makes You Radioactive and Dangerous to Others

Once you have had EBRT, you will not become permanently or even temporarily radioactive. This means that you can still hang around with your friends, their babies and children, and everyone else, and you can also go through airport security with no problem. However, with brachytherapy, if you receive a high dosage of radiation, then you may be temporarily radioactive, which is why your doctor will deliver this therapy to you in a controlled environment, often in a hospital room. Your doctor will tell you about any safety measures that you will need to take while in the hospital. Once you are discharged from the hospital, then your radioactive quotient should be nonexistent.

Myth: Radiation Therapy Destroys All Your Skin

Radiation therapy may burn and irritate your skin at the site of the radiation (your chest), but you will recover. Think of it as a really bad sunburn. The radiation still penetrates the skin and can cause burning, itching, and pain.

Myth: Radiation Makes You Bald

Unless it's your scalp that's irradiated, you won't experience any hair loss from your radiation treatments for breast cancer. You may lose your hair if you have radiation *and* chemotherapy within the same time frame, but if so, it was the *chemo* that caused the hair loss and not the radiation. The radiation for breast cancer is very targeted.

Myth: Radiation Kills Cancer Cells So They Can Never Come Back

This is a myth that I really wish were true! Radiation treatments are very powerful but are delivered to only one area of your body. But unfortunately, even when radiation wipes out your current cancer cells, it is still possible to develop breast cancer again sometime down the road in the future. That's why it's very important to be vigilant with your medical checkups once your current cancer therapy has been completed.

Myth: Radiation Therapy Is Painful

The radiation treatments themselves are not painful, although the side effects later may cause some irritation or pain. During your treatments, you may feel nothing at all or you could feel a slight feeling of warmth, one that is not painful.

Newer Forms of Radiation Therapy

Radiologists are always trying to improve their treatments for breast cancer as well as other forms of cancer. For example, accelerated partial-breast irradiation (APBI) is a type of radiation that treats the patient with a higher dose of radiation for a shorter period of time compared to other forms of radiation therapy. APBI may be given both internally or externally and may be given twice a day for five days, after which treatment is complete.[14] Doctors disagree on whether this type of radiation is better than EBRT or brachytherapy. They also disagree on the effects on your skin, with some saying you'll have a better outcome and some insisting the outcome is worse with APBI. Because of its newness, this type of radiation therapy is only available at some major medical centers.

Notes

1. American Cancer Society Cancer Action Network, "Breast Cancer in African American Women," Undated, http://www.acscan.org/content/wp-content/uploads/2014/09/AAwomenandBC.pdf (accessed September 12, 2016).

2. Michael J. Hassett et al., "Variation in Breast Cancer Care Quality in New York and California Based on Race/Ethnicity and Medicaid Enrollment," *Cancer* 122 (2016): 420–431.

3. Jean Wright et al., "Prospective Evaluation of Radiation-Induced Skin Toxicity in a Race/Ethnically Diverse Breast Cancer Population," *Cancer Medicine* 5, no. 3 (2016): 454–464.

4. American Cancer Society, *Breast Cancer*, Atlanta, GA, September 13, 2016, http://www.cancer.org/acs/groups/cid/documents/webcontent/003090-pdf.pdf (accessed September 19, 2016).

5. California Department of Health Services, Cancer Detection and Treatment Branch, *A Woman's Guide to Breast Cancer Treatment*, Sacramento, CA, January 2016.

6. Grace L. Smith et al., "Utilization and Outcomes of Breast Brachytherapy in Younger Women," *International Journal of Radiation Oncology* 93 (2015): 91–101.

7. American Cancer Society, "Radiation Therapy for Breast Cancer," September 13, 2016, http://www.cancer.org/cancer/breastcancer/detailedguide/breast-cancer-treating-radiation (accessed September 18, 2016).

8. Ibid.

9. Ibid.

10. California Department of Health Services, Cancer Detection and Treatment Branch, *A Woman's Guide to Breast Cancer Treatment*, Sacramento, CA, January 2016.

11. National Cancer Institute, "Fatigue (PDQ®)–Patient Version," May 7, 2015, https://www.cancer.gov/about-cancer/treatment/side-effects/fatigue/fatigue-pdq (accessed September 19, 2016).

12. Leanna J. Standish et al., "Immune Deficits in Breast Cancer Patients after Radiotherapy," *Journal of the Society for Integrative Oncology* 6, no. 3 (2008): 110–121.

13. Mayo Clinic, "Low Blood Cell Counts: Side Effect of Cancer Treatment," http://www.mayoclinic.org/diseases-conditions/cancer/in-depth/cancer-treatment/art-20046192 (accessed August 6, 2016).

14. California Department of Health Services, Cancer Detection and Treatment Branch, *A Woman's Guide to Breast Cancer Treatment*, Sacramento, CA, January 2016.

CHAPTER EIGHT

Chemotherapy, Anti-Estrogen (Endocrine) Therapy, Combined Therapies, and Emerging Treatments

With breast cancer, often one type of therapy (surgery, radiation, endocrine therapy, or chemotherapy) is not considered enough treatment to adequately combat the disease. The reason for this is that the breast cancer cells may also be present in areas of the body away from the breast. In addition, different treatments have varying targets in the cancer cells. Ultimately, how these different therapies are prescribed to a given patient also goes to the heart of personalized medicine. As a result, your doctor may recommend different combinations of therapies to different patients because the tumors are not considered the same in all women with breast cancer. Each woman is unique, and the treatment that you may need to treat your breast cancer may be a completely different treatment regimen than what I needed to treat my cancer or that another woman needs to treat her breast cancer. In this chapter, I talk about chemotherapy, endocrine therapy, targeted therapy, and other emerging treatments that are designed to destroy those breast cancer cells.

Talking about Chemotherapy

Chemotherapy, also known as cytotoxic therapy, refers to special medications that you are given to rid your body of those nasty cancer cells by killing them. These treatments either destroy the cancer cells directly or prevent them from continuing to divide and multiply. These drugs also result in some collateral damage to the normal cells. However, the effect on the normal cells is fully reversible in most cases, depending on the type of cancer and the treatment plan of the medical oncologist. As mentioned in the chapter on radiation therapy (Chapter Seven), chemotherapy may be given by itself or in concert with surgery, radiation therapy, or other treatments for breast cancer.

It's also important for you to know that chemotherapy may be given at any stage of cancer, so don't assume that if the doctor orders chemo, then this must mean you have an advanced stage of cancer. It may mean that, but it also may not. Having said that, however, it is much less common to use chemotherapy in the very early stages of the disease. If you're in doubt, ask questions! It's good and even imperative to ask your doctor questions about the stage and type of the cancer, so you help ensure the best outcome possible.

Unfortunately, the side effects from chemotherapy drugs often can be pretty tough for your healthy cells (and you) to cope with. It's not just the hair loss and the other side effects, like nausea and vomiting. It's also the exhausted feeling that you may get that's like you just ran a marathon, when all you did was get out of bed. I was able to withstand radiation treatments and still go to work without a problem. But when I had chemotherapy, it wiped me out, and I had to take a leave of absence from my job as a senior analyst. I was flat on my back, and for me, it felt like an effort to just breathe. I knew that it was necessary for me to have chemotherapy to get rid of the cancer, so I stayed the course, and the chemo did its job. However, as I have said throughout this book, treatments affect people differently, so you may have a very different response to chemotherapy than I experienced.

When Chemotherapy Is Used

Chemotherapy may be used at different phases of treatment. For example, it may be used before surgery for the purpose of helping to shrink a large tumor. This is called preoperative or neoadjuvant chemotherapy. Chemotherapy may also be used *after* surgery to decrease the risk of a recurrence of the breast cancer in the future, which is referred to as adjuvant therapy. Chemotherapy may also be used instead of surgery when breast cancer has spread to other parts of the body. Sometimes chemotherapy is used to decrease a woman's pain by shrinking the tumor, as when a large tumor presses down and causes pain.

Often administered in cycles of treatment that are separated by one to three weeks or some other period determined by the oncologist,

POVERTY AND BLACK RACE LINKED TO DELAYS IN CHEMO

Poverty is bad no matter what the race of a person is, but if that person is a black woman with breast cancer who needs chemotherapy, it may be especially onerous, based on recent research. In a study reported in 2012 in *Ethnicity & Disease,* the researchers found that black women on Medicaid who had breast cancer were twice as likely as white women on Medicaid to face treatment delays with chemotherapy.[1]

In this study, the researchers drew their data from subjects in the New Jersey State Cancer Registry and the New Jersey Medicaid Research files. There were 237 black subjects and 485 white subjects, and all the subjects were on Medicaid. The study subjects were 20–64 years old and all were diagnosed with early-stage breast cancer.

The black women were significantly more likely than the white women in the study to have chemotherapy delays of three months or longer after their surgery. The black women were also more likely to experience delays in receiving chemotherapy after radiation. (These treatment delays were not seen with other forms of treatment.)

It was unclear why the black women experienced such a delay regarding chemotherapy but the researchers noted that the black subjects were more likely to be younger and unmarried than were the white Medicaid subjects. It might be interesting to study whether the unmarried black women who experienced delayed treatment had young children at home and if that factor had any effect on their delayed chemotherapy. With surgery, treatment was not delayed, but it may be possible to find temporary backup child care for a major procedure such as breast cancer surgery. After the surgery, the patient recovers. In contrast, chemotherapy may cause continuous severe sickness throughout treatment, and possibly would mitigate against the ill parent taking care of a child. It's one possible reason to explore, and there are many other potential reasons why black women in the study experienced treatment delays with chemotherapy.

Because they often face more aggressive and faster-growing forms of breast cancer, as discussed in other chapters of this book, it's important for black women to receive treatment as soon as possible after their diagnosis. When this doesn't happen, researchers need to find out WHY it doesn't happen, so that, whatever the underlying problems are, they can be resolved. We know there's a problem. We just don't know what the cause of the problem is, although theories proliferate. (Poverty, lack of education, and many other possible reasons have been demonstrated to be factors in the problem of worse prognoses for black women, but we don't know if they are the cause of the problem.)

[1] Bijal A. Balasubramanian et al., "Black Medicaid Beneficiaries Experience Breast Cancer Treatment Delays More Frequently than Whites," *Ethnicity & Disease* 22 (Summer 2012): 288–294.

chemotherapy involves several cycles of treatment. There is a rest period after each cycle to give your body's healthy cells a chance to recover from the effects of chemotherapy. Chemotherapy may be given for three to six months or for a shorter or longer period, because each person's case is different. If your doctor recommends that you receive chemo, be sure to ask how long the entire treatment will last, how many cycles of treatment are recommended, and how long will the rest period be between the cycles of treatment. (I also list other questions to ask about chemotherapy later in this chapter.)

Combinations of Chemotherapies

Chemotherapy may be given as one medication alone or it may be administered in combination with other forms of chemotherapy. For example, one combination uses Adriamycin (doxorubicin hydrochloride) with Cytoxan (cyclophosphamide), which is subsequently followed with Taxol (paclitaxel). This form of therapy is abbreviated as AC-T or called the AC-T regimen. Another combination uses Adriamycin and Cytoxan, followed by Taxol and then Herceptin (trastuzumab). This is called the AC-TH regimen or the AC-T-T regimen.[1] If your doctor believes a combination therapy approach is right for you, he will tell you about it and explain why it would be best for your case.

Side Effects of Chemotherapy

There are some difficult side effects that many women experience from chemotherapy for breast cancer. The chemo is used to kill your cancer cells, but it can also often upset your entire body considerably. The reason for this is because chemotherapy is a systemic kind of therapy affecting your whole body, rather than a localized type of treatment like radiation or surgery, which concentrates on one part of the body. Be also aware that different drugs can lead to different side effects. In addition, the intensity of the side effects to the same drug can vary considerably from woman to woman, and this is partly based on genetic makeup. This means that a drug that may make your friend extremely sick may cause you only minor side effects.

The primary side effects that you may experience with chemotherapy include the following, and I will elaborate further on some of them in this section.

- Anemia
- Low white blood cell counts
- Low blood platelet counts
- Infections
- Nausea and vomiting
- Fatigue
- Loss of appetite and weight loss
- Damage to the ovaries
- Decreased mental function
- Hair loss
- Mouth sores
- Diarrhea or constipation
- Difficulty with short- or long-term memory
- An early menopause
- Infertility
- Heart damage
- Nerve disease/pain (neuropathy)
- Bone damage (osteoporosis)

Nausea and Vomiting

Nausea and vomiting are chemotherapy side effects that may occur shortly after you start treatment or this problem could occur later on in treatment. Nowadays there are several medications and combinations of medications that are very effective in preventing the nausea and vomiting that may be associated with chemotherapy. Some examples are Zofran (ondansetron), Compazine (prochlorperazine), Valium (lorazepam), and Decadron (dexamethasone), as well as other medications.

Fatigue

Fatigue is a very common side effect of chemotherapy. Fatigue may also accumulate over time and get worse during the course of therapy. Some people are so tired that it feels like an effort to pick up a spoon or a fork to eat a meal, while the fatigue is much milder in other individuals. You'll still need to eat something to survive, of course, so pick up that spoon or fork anyway. Take naps as needed, but be sure to also push yourself to exercise by taking a walk once a day. Your body won't thank you right away, but it will later on. Be sure to tell your doctor about the extent of your fatigue, so he can make any necessary adjustments to your therapy.

Hair Loss

Hair loss is very common with chemotherapy and it varies with the use of different drugs. Some people get ready for the hair loss by shaving all their hair off or by getting a very short haircut. Others buy wigs. Note that your health insurance may cover the cost of a wig, which is sometimes also known as a "hair cranial prosthesis" by insurance companies. They love their fancy phrases!

After your cancer treatments end completely, your hair may start to grow back within a few months. When hair does grow back, it may be a different color and/or texture. So your curly black hair may turn gray or white and could be much straighter or curlier than it was before. It could also be finer or coarser than before you had the chemotherapy.

During the time frame when you have no hair, be sure to protect your head. Wear a wig or a scarf to cover your head to protect it from the sun or from the cold.

IF YOU ARE STILL FERTILE, DON'T ASSUME YOU CAN'T GET PREGNANT WHILE RECEIVING CHEMOTHERAPY

Chemotherapy may and often does reduce a woman's fertility, especially in women over 40 years old. But never assume that it's impossible to get pregnant while receiving chemotherapy. You could end up with a distressing surprise! (Chemotherapy is not good for growing fetuses.) Instead, if you are normally capable of pregnancy and if you are still having sexual intercourse during this time, be sure to use a barrier type of contraception (like condoms, a diaphragm, and spermicide) while receiving chemotherapy.

Loss of Appetite and Weight Loss

So many people are overweight or obese in our society that it may seem like a very good thing to lose some weight. But when the weight loss is involuntary and if it is a result of the appetite loss caused by cancer treatment, this is not desirable. Be sure to tell your doctor if you are experiencing a poor appetite and a significant weight loss (more than 10 pounds), and she may be able to suggest medications that could help during this time. Also, be sure to drink plenty of fluids. You don't need to add dehydration to your list of problems!

Damage to the Ovaries

Some chemotherapy drugs may damage the ovaries and some women may experience early menopause-like symptoms, such as hot flashes, night sweats, mood swings, and vaginal dryness. If you still menstruate, your periods may become irregular or they may stop altogether with chemotherapy and not return when treatment has been completed. The older that the woman receiving chemotherapy is, the more likely this side effect will occur. The woman who goes through a medically induced menopause may be unable to become pregnant. However, many younger women freeze their eggs before treatment with the hope of having an in vitro fertilization procedure to have a child later on.

It's best to avoid pregnancy while you are receiving chemotherapy because chemotherapy drugs can cause birth defects in early pregnancy.

Decreased Mental Function

Some women report that they can't think as well during chemotherapy treatment, and this side effect even has its own name, "chemo brain." This side effect causes difficulty in concentration and may also affect your memory as well. It may take some time to recover from chemo brain, if it happens to you, and experts say that the effects of chemo brain may last as long as several years after chemotherapy treatment.[2]

Heart and Cardiovascular Damage

Chemotherapy drugs can be harmful to the heart and the patient should be carefully followed. According to some researchers, survivors of breast cancer who have received chemotherapy have an elevated risk for cardiovascular diseases, such as hypertension, heart arrhythmia, congestive heart failure, and thromboembolic events (blood clots).[3] It is clear that regular checkups are important for the current breast cancer patient as well as the breast cancer survivor.

Neuropathy

Nerve damage, especially peripheral neuropathy, may be caused by chemotherapy drugs, according to the American Cancer Society.[4] When nerve damage occurs after the use of chemotherapy drugs, this disorder is known as chemotherapy-induced peripheral neuropathy (CIPN). The peripheral nerves are important because they control arm and leg movements and also carry sensations back to the brain. In addition, the peripheral nerves control both the bowel and the bladder. Some symptoms of CIPN are as follows:

- Burning feeling
- Pain that may be constant or intermittent
- Paresthesia (feelings of "pins and needles")
- An inability to feel pressure, heat, or cold or an increased sensitivity
- Difficulty picking up and holding things
- Problems with balance
- Difficulty with tripping while walking
- Impaired body reflexes
- Difficulty with urination

According to the American Cancer Society, the following medications may cause CIPN:

- Platinum drugs such as Platinol (cisplatin), Panuplatin (carboplatin), and Elaxatin (oxaliplatin)
- All taxanes, including Taxol (paclitaxel), Taxotere (docetaxel), and Jevtana (carbazitaxel)
- Ixempra (ixabepilone)
- Plant alkaloids, including vinblastine (Velban), Marqibo (vincristine), Navelbine (vinorelbine), and etopoxide (VP-16)
- Belcade (bortexomib)
- Kyprolis (carfilzomib
- Revlimid (lenalidomide)
- Pomalyst (pomalidomide)
- Halaven (Eribulin)[5]

Bone Damage

Chemotherapy drugs can lead to a decrease in bone density and to osteoporosis, and the onset may be rapid. This is why women with breast cancer and their physicians should keep bone health in mind. Experts say that often osteoporosis is a "silent" disease because it remains undetected unless a woman suffers a fracture. Other factors that may increase the risk of osteoporosis include the following:

- Age over 50 years
- A small and thin body frame
- An early onset of menopause
- A previous history of a bone fracture
- The use of tobacco
- The use of alcohol[6]

Some medications increase the risk for osteoporosis, including the following drugs:

- Aromatase inhibitors (chemotherapy)
- Proton pump inhibitors (for stomach problems)
- Some antidepressants
- Anticonvulsants (antiseizure medications)
- Anticoagulants (blood thinners)
- Glucocorticoids (some anti-inflammatory medications)[7]

Questions to Ask Your Doctor about Your Chemotherapy

Of course, you can and should come up with your own questions about chemotherapy to ask your doctor. But the National Cancer Institute offers some questions for you to consider:

- Why do I need chemotherapy?
- What is the goal of this chemotherapy?
- What are the expected benefits of chemotherapy?
- What are the risks?
- Are there other ways to treat my cancer?
- What is the standard care for my type of cancer?
- How many cycles of chemotherapy will I get?

- Where will I go to receive treatment
- How long will each treatment last?
- What side effects can I expect right away?
- What side effects can I expect later?
- How long will these side effects last?
- When should I call my doctor or nurse about these side effects?
- Is it okay to have sex during chemotherapy if I want to?
- Will all the side effects go away when treatment is over?[8]

What You Need to Know about Anti-Estrogen/Endocrine Therapy

Endocrine therapy is sometimes called "hormone therapy" because it is therapy that directly affects specific hormones (and endocrine glands are responsible for hormone production). The most common form of this treatment targets the female sex hormone estrogen and is used for treating an initial breast cancer tumor as well as with a breast cancer recurrence.[9] These drugs are often given in the pill form (e.g., Nolvadex, or tamoxifen), but they may also be given by injection.

Endocrine therapy works by either lowering the estrogen levels in your body or by blocking their effect on the cancer cells and other normal cells. Some endocrine therapies that block estrogen are also known as estrogen blockers or anti-estrogens. This treatment may be used before or after surgery, depending on your individual case and what your doctor recommends. Sometimes more than one form of endocrine therapy may be used over a period of several years.

Before you start endocrine therapy, be sure to tell your doctor about all other medications you are taking, because some drugs may interfere with or impede the effects of your endocrine therapy. For example, according to the National Cancer Institute, common antidepressants in the selective serotonin reuptake inhibitor (SSRI) class can interfere with the use of Nolvadex (tamoxifen). SSRIs include such drugs as Prozac (fluoxetine) or Effexor (venlafaxine). If antidepressants are needed, the doctor may wish to switch the patient to another medication that is less likely to weaken the Nolvadex (or other endocrine therapy) or that is a weaker inhibitor. Other medications that may also weaken the effect of endocrine therapy include diphenhydramine, an antihistamine, and also quinidine (Quinaglute, Quinidex), a drug that treats abnormal heart rhythms. Interestingly, this drug also has a very different use—it is also used to treat malaria![10]

ENDOCRINE THERAPY FOR CANCER IS NOT THE SAME AS HORMONE REPLACEMENT THERAPY

Hormone replacement therapy (HRT) is the administration to a menopausal woman of hormones like estrogen or progesterone that have been specifically prescribed to decrease the symptoms of menopause, such as hot flashes, night sweats, and mood swings. In the 20th century, many menopausal women were routinely prescribed HRT, which was seen as a sort of "fountain of youth"; however, researchers found that this therapy increased the risk for diseases like breast cancer. Very simply, estrogen can make cancer grow. In very stark contrast to HRT, there is a different type of endocrine (hormone) therapy that is given to some women with breast cancer to *decrease* their sex hormone levels so that the cancer will be starved out from the estrogen that it needs to grow. If you hear the phrase "hormone therapy," and you're not sure what is meant, then be sure to ask!

Hormone-Blocking Drugs

The most commonly known medication in the category of hormone-blocking drugs is Nolvadex (tamoxifen), and this medication can be used in either premenopausal or postmenopausal women with breast cancer. Another medication in this category is Fareston (toremifene), and it may be used when breast cancer has spread beyond the breast. The medications that block the estrogen receptors that are found in breast cancer cells are also sometimes called selective estrogen receptor modulators (SERMs). These drugs are used only in women with hormone receptor–positive breast cancer. These drugs are usually taken as a pill. Faslodex (fulvestrant) is a third hormone-blocking medication, but it is not a SERM. Doctors may choose this drug when Nolvadex is no longer working or the woman is no longer responding to a drug in the aromatase inhibitor class of medications, a specific category of endocrine therapy drugs that is discussed next. This drug is also used to treat metastatic breast cancer.[11]

Aromatase Inhibitors: Estrogen-Lowering Drugs

Aromatase inhibitors (AIs) are medications in a category of drugs that block the production of estradiol, another female hormone. These drugs are used only in women who have already gone through menopause, and as of this writing in 2016, they include Arimedex (anastrozole), Aromasin (exemestane), and Femara (letrozole). This type of endocrine therapy is usually used in postmenopausal women who have breast cancer.[12] Important note is if you are taking or have previously taken a medication in this drug category, then you should be sure to receive a bone density test, because the drug can thin out the bones, leading to osteopenia or, in the worst case, osteoporosis. Women with osteoporosis who fall are more likely than others to suffer bone fractures.

Side Effects of Endocrine Therapy

As with all cancer treatment therapies, there are side effects with endocrine therapy, and they largely include the effects of menopause as well as a few other adverse effects. Be sure to ask your doctor about the specific side effects of the medication that she prescribes.

In general, these side effects may include some or more of the following:

- Weight gain
- Hot flashes
- Mood swings
- Vaginal dryness
- Thinning hair
- Headaches
- Cataracts in the eyes
- Increased cholesterol levels
- Joint pain and stiffness
- Heart problems
- Upset stomach
- Weakening of the bones

Ovarian Ablation/Hormone Stopping

Sometimes the surgical removal of the ovaries is recommended to block the body's natural production of estrogen, since estrogen can make breast cancer grow faster. This surgery is known as an oophorectomy, and it is a permanent and irreversible change that will make the woman infertile and menopausal. However, more commonly, estrogen production can be blocked with luteinizing hormone-releasing (LHRH) analogs, which are medications given by injections (once every month or every three months) and which temporarily cause the symptoms of menopause. Once the drug wears off, normal estrogen production usually will resume. The

---

AMONG BLACK WOMEN, ADHERENCE TO HORMONE THERAPY IS TIED TO INCOME

In a study of more than 10,000 women treated with hormone therapy for early-stage breast cancer, Dawn L. Hershman and colleagues found that 24 percent of the patients were nonadherent, which means that they didn't comply with the treatment plan, either by discontinuing the drug altogether or by not following the medication regimen. In this study, there were about 8,000 white subjects with breast cancer, and about 1,000 black subjects, and the balance of the women were Hispanic, Asian, or "other." All the subjects were aged 50 years or older. The researchers determined the women's medication adherence by whether the medication was refilled over time—or not—as well as by the number of endocrine therapy pills that were dispensed.

The researchers found that the black subjects were less likely to be compliant with the endocrine therapy than the subjects of other races, and when household net worth was added in as a variable, the researchers found that low levels of net worth and being black also correlated with being nonadherent with medication therapy. It is possible that the out-of-pocket costs of the medication for the patients of lower income directly affected their compliance with endocrine therapy. One reason to think this was that the researchers found that adherence rates increased when the patients were switched to generic drugs from brand-name drugs. Since generics are invariably less costly than brand-name drugs, this finding also indicates that cost may affect medication compliance or adherence.[1] The researchers also noted that women of high income levels were more likely to be compliant with endocrine therapy treatment than were women of low income, regardless of race. This study identified an important problem that needs to be considered by doctors who recommend endocrine therapy for their black patients, as well as their low-income patients of any race, because nonadherence with treatment can affect the outcome of the women's breast cancer.[2]

[1]Dawn L. Hershman et al., "Household Net Worth, Social Disparities, and Hormonal Therapy Adherence among Women with Early-Stage Breast Cancer," *Journal of Clinical Oncology* 33 (2015): 1053–1059.

[2]Ibid.

most common LHRH drugs used to treat breast cancer are Zoladex (goserelin) and Lupron (leuprolide). These drugs may be used by themselves or in concert with other hormone therapy.

Targeted Therapy

The human epidermal genetic factor receptor 2 (HER2) is a molecule on the surface of the breast cancer, which facilitates growth and the multiplication of the cancer cells and their spread. Among patients who are HER2 positive (20–30 percent of all women with breast cancer), there are four major drugs that are used for therapy as of this writing: Herceptin (trastuzumab), Perjeta (pertuzumab), Tykerb (lapatinib), and Kadcyla (ado-trastuzumab emtansine). Herceptin is the most commonly known of the targeted therapies in breast cancer, and it is used alongside chemotherapy in HER2-positive women.

Herceptin is in the category of medications that are known as monoclonal antibodies. They are medications that were molecularly engineered and synthesized to target the HER2 molecule. When Herceptin is used in early cancer, it is often administered for at least a year. If the cancer is more advanced, it may be used for as long as it appears to be effective. Herceptin is administered intravenously.[13]

Perjeta (pertuzumab) is another monoclonal antibody and it may be given alongside Herceptin as well as with chemotherapy to treat advanced cancer. This drug is also administered intravenously. Kadcyla (ado-trastuzumab emtansine) is also used to treat advanced breast cancer and it is administered intravenously.[14]

CONSIDERING A MEDICATION FOR BONE HEALTH

Chemotherapy and other medications used to treat breast cancer may lead to a significantly decreased level of bone density. In my own case, I am taking a medication called Arimedix (anastrozole), and a major side effect is osteoporosis, as well as bone pain and night sweats. Arimedix is a medication that is given to some postmenopausal women and I will be on this therapy for another three years for a total of five years. Arimedix is given after chemotherapy or in the place of chemo, such as in my case. A medically induced osteoporosis is an important issue for all women with breast cancer to keep in mind, because osteoporosis can lead to serious bone fractures.

Tykerb (laptinib) is a targeted drug that is in the category of medications known as kinase inhibitors. It is given as a pill and used in advanced cancer, and is often used alongside either chemotherapy or hormone therapy.

Targeted Therapies for Hormone Receptor–Positive Breast Cancer

When the breast cancer is known to be hormone receptor positive, the physician may treat with other newer medications such as Ibrance (palbociclib) or Afinitor (everolimus). Afinitor is only used with women who have already undergone menopause. Ibrance is often given along with hormone therapy drugs in the aromatase inhibitor class.[15]

Heart damage is a possible risk with targeted therapy for HER2 breast cancer, particularly when it is administered with chemotherapy medications that also increase the risk for heart disease, such as Ellence (epirubicin) or Adriamycin (doxorubicin). Thus, periodic echocardiograms are needed when these medications are taken.[16]

Side Effects with Targeted Therapy

As with all cancer therapies, there are side effects with targeted therapy, and they may include nausea, fever, and chills, similar to the symptoms of having the flu. Each different drug has its own set of potential side effects, and you should ask your doctor what they may be. Remember, not everyone experiences these side effects, and also, if you do experience side effects, they may be mild, moderate, or severe. Always tell your doctor about any side effects that you may experience subsequent to targeted therapy (or any other type of therapy for breast cancer). When used along with chemotherapy, targeted therapy may cause infection or anemia.[17]

The National Cancer Institute recommends you ask your doctor the following questions if she recommends targeted therapy for you. Note that these same questions may be used to ask your doctor about hormone therapy.

- What drugs will I be taking?
- When will treatment start and when will it end?
- How often will I receive treatment?
- Where will I receive treatment?
- How will we know that the treatment is working?
- What side effects should I tell you about?[18]

Emerging Therapies

Some researchers are testing possible vaccines against breast cancer, and there is also an array of other tools that may be used in the future to effectively target and destroy the cancer cells. In an entirely different area of study, one young researcher found a way to effectively target bacterial cells so that bacterial infections that were impervious to antibiotics were destroyed in mice by introducing a substance known as a nano-polymer, a tiny organic synthesized material.[19] Perhaps such a technique could be adapted to target cancer cells at some future point. However, as of this writing, immunotherapy has not shown enough encouraging data, and research is ongoing.

Clinical Studies

You should always ask your doctor whether there is a clinical study or trial that is suitable for you. A clinical study is a research study that is performed by experts in the field, and it is also an opportunity to obtain a treatment or medication that is not available to the general public because it hasn't been approved by the Food and Drug Administration (FDA) yet. The researchers often need volunteers to participate in the study. Studies may also test new methods of screening, diagnosis, treatment, or prevention of breast cancer or other forms of cancer. Yet often black women do not consider joining clinical trials.

There are four primary phases of a clinical study. Phase I is a test of the best way to administer a brand new treatment. Phase II clinical trials are designed to test whether a specific treatment is actually effective in treating a particular disease. Phase III clinical studies compare the results of individuals using the new treatment to the results of those using the standard treatment for the disease. Last, Phase IV clinical trials test the treatment on thousands of individuals after the treatment has been approved by the FDA and is in use by patients in the population. The purpose of Phase IV clinical studies is to check for any side effects that were not previously discovered in Phase III trials.

Every patient with cancer is strongly encouraged to enroll in a clinical trial. Clinical trials offer a high standard of medical care and also allow an opportunity to access new and promising drugs. None of the drugs medical science has at this time will cure advanced breast cancer, although they would allow long-term survival. We need drugs that would cure this disease even in its most advanced form of disease; and therefore, clinical trials are very important.

The "downside" of a clinical study is that some subjects do not receive the new drug for the purposes of comparison with the subjects who do receive it. This means that you could be in the group that does not receive the therapy or drug, or the "placebo" group, and you won't know which group you are in because the researchers are not allowed to tell you. In addition, even if you do receive the new therapy, it may not be effective. On the plus side, you may receive the drug and it may be very effective. When there are no good options to try, a clinical study may be the right choice for you. Ask your doctor for more information about clinical studies and whether she recommends that you join one.

You may search for current and past clinical studies on breast cancer and other medication topics on the Internet at the FDA website at this online location: https://clinicaltrials.gov/ct2/search/advanced.

Notes

1. National Cancer Institute, *NCI Dictionary of Cancer Terms*, Bethesda, MD, Undated, https://www.cancer.gov/publications/dictionaries/cancer-terms, (accessed September 30, 2016).

2. American Cancer Society, *Breast Cancer.* Atlanta, GA, September 13, 2016, http://www.cancer.org/acs/groups/cid/documents/webcontent/003090-pdf.pdf (accessed September 19, 2016).

3. Balazs I. Bodai and Philip Tuso, "Breast Cancer Survivorship: A Comprehensive Review of Long-Term Medical Issues and Lifestyle Recommendations," *The Permanente Journal* 19, no. 2 (Spring 2015): 48–75.

4. American Cancer Society, *Peripheral Neuropathy Caused by Chemotherapy*, May 10, 2016, http://www.cancer.org/acs/groups/cid/documents/webcontent/002 908-pdf.pdf (accessed December 12, 2016).

5. Ibid.

6. Balazs I. Bodai and Philip Tuso, "Breast Cancer Survivorship: A Comprehensive Review of Long-Term Medical Issues and Lifestyle Recommendations," *The Permanente Journal* 19, no. 2 (Spring 2015): 48–75.

7. Ibid.

8. National Cancer Institute, *Chemotherapy and You*, Bethesda, MD, 2011, https://www.cancer.gov/publications/patient-education/chemotherapy-and-you .pdf (accessed September 27, 2016).

9. California Department of Health Services, Cancer Detection and Treatment Branch, *A Woman's Guide to Breast Cancer Treatment*, January 2016.

10. National Cancer Institute, "Hormone Therapy for Breast Cancer," August 2, 2012, http://www.cancer.gov/types/breast/breast-hormone-therapy-fact-sheet (accessed September 30, 2016).

11. American Cancer Society, *Breast Cancer*, Atlanta, GA, September 13, 2016, http://www.cancer.org/acs/groups/cid/documents/webcontent/003090-pdf.pdf (accessed September 19, 2016).

12. California Department of Health Services, Cancer Detection and Treatment Branch, *A Woman's Guide to Breast Cancer Treatment*. Sacramento, CA, January 2016.

13. American Cancer Society, "Targeted Therapy for Breast Cancer," September 13, 2016, http://www.cancer.org/cancer/breastcancer/detailedguide/breast-cancer-treating-targeted-therapy (accessed September 30, 2016).

14. Ibid.

15. Ibid.

16. Ibid.

17. California Department of Health Services, Cancer Detection and Treatment Branch, *A Woman's Guide to Breast Cancer Treatment*, Sacramento, CA, January 2016.

18. National Cancer Institute, *What You Need to Know about Breast Cancer*, Bethesda, MD, 2012, http://www.cancer.gov/publications/patient-education/wyntk-breast.pdf (accessed August 28, 2016).

19. Fiona McDonald, "The Science World Is Freaking Out over This 25-Year-Old's Answer to Antibiotic Resistance," *Science Alert*, September 26, 2016, http://www.sciencealert.com/the-science-world-s-freaking-out-over-this-25-year-old-s-solution-to-antibiotic-resistance (accessed September 30, 2016).

CHAPTER NINE

Watching Out for Other Forms of Cancer

In addition to having high risks for breast cancer, black women also have a higher risk than women of other races and ethnicities for other types of cancer, particularly lung cancer, cervical cancer, and colorectal cancer. I will cover the signs, symptoms, and important facts to know about each form of cancer in this chapter. I am also going to include thyroid cancer in this discussion, since I developed thyroid cancer myself.

In looking at black women in general and at all forms of cancer, the American Cancer Society says that the death rate is 14 percent higher for black women with cancer than for white women with cancer. This is partly because blacks have a disproportionately higher rate of other diseases, which also affect survival, such as heart disease. It is also true that the overall life expectancy is lower for blacks, such as 78.4 years for black women compared to 81.4 years for white women.[1] According to some researchers, this disparity between the death rates for black and white women with breast cancer has occurred since the 1970s.[2] It is also possible that there are racial disparities between black women and white women in terms of their outcomes with other forms of cancer, just as I have demonstrated throughout this book with breast cancer.

Breast cancer is the most commonly diagnosed form of cancer among black women, but it is lung cancer that represents the greatest number of deaths from cancer among black women, or 22 percent of all cancer deaths in 2016. Breast cancer represents the next leading cause of cancer death for black women (19 percent) followed by colorectal cancer (10 percent). I realize this is distressing data and I don't want you to think that everyone who develops one of these forms of cancer cannot recover, because that's just not true. There are about 1.3 million black male and female cancer survivors in the United States today.[3]

Routine Checkups Often Identify Existing Common Cancers

Often routine checkups and tests can detect cancer. For example, your gynecologist will check you for cervical cancer with the pap smear, which is a simple test performed during a routine gynecological examination. The colonoscopy is a test that frequently detects colorectal cancer if it is present. The colonoscopy is a more invasive test than the pap smear, and most people hate the preparation part more than the actual test because the preparation for the test causes severe diarrhea to completely empty the colon. This is done so that when the doctor visualizes the inside, it will be clean and easy to inspect. A sigmoidoscopy is another test for colorectal cancer but it provides a more limited view of the colon. Some doctors have said that a sigmoidoscopy is like having a mammogram of one breast.

MAINTAIN A COPY OF YOUR MEDICAL RECORDS

The National Cancer Institute says that individuals who have had cancer in the past should ask their oncologist for a written copy of their records. This is important information that can be shared with other doctors in the future. You may wish to keep these records in a binder or a special folder. Keep the following information in your records:

- Your date of diagnosis of cancer
- The type of cancer for which you were treated
- Pathology reports that describe the type and stage of the cancer
- Places and dates of specific treatments, such as details of surgeries, sites and total amounts of radiation received, and names and doses of chemotherapy and all other drugs used to treat the cancer
- Key lab reports, X-ray reports, CT scan reports, and MRI reports
- A list of cancer signs that you should watch out for and the possible long-term effects of treatment
- Contact information for all the health professionals who were involved in your treatment and follow-up care
- Information on any problems that occurred during your treatment[1]

[1]National Cancer Institute, *Facing Forward: Life after Cancer Treatment*, Bethesda, MD, May 2014, https://www.cancer.gov/publications/patient-education/life-after-treatment .pdf (accessed October 1, 2016).

Having one type of cancer, like breast cancer, doesn't necessarily mean that you are more prone to having another type of cancer. But it also doesn't mean that you are safe from other common cancers either, so be sure to have regular physical examinations and to alert your doctor if you have any symptoms that should be checked out.

It's also true that sometimes cancer from one part of the body migrates to another area. If breast cancer cells travel to another part of the body, it is still breast cancer no matter where the cells are located in your body, and the same is true for other forms of cancer. When cancer starts in one place and then lodges elsewhere, such as the lung, this is referred to as a secondary tumor. Your oncologist will advise you on the best treatment for this secondary tumor.

Lung Cancer

Lung cancer is the leading cause of death from cancer among black women in the United States. In 2016, an estimated 11,010 black women were diagnosed with lung cancer. Among black women, lung cancer is the second most diagnosed form of cancer after breast cancer. An estimated 32 percent of black women diagnosed with cancer in the period 2008–2012 had breast cancer, followed by 11 percent with lung cancer and 9 percent with colorectal cancer.[4]

There are two primary types of lung cancer, small cell lung cancer and non–small cell lung cancer. Of these, the small cell lung cancer, which is less common, has a worse prognosis.

Lung cancer continues to be a problem in the United States, largely because too many people still smoke cigarettes. Smoking is the single most preventable cause of death for lung cancer, and among women, at least 76 percent of lung cancer deaths are smoking-related.[5] Secondhand smoke—being around others who smoke—can also cause lung cancer.

If you smoke, then you should receive regular physical examinations so that if you do develop lung cancer, it will be detected and treated. The best choice is to stop smoking.

Signs and Symptoms of Lung Cancer

Women with lung cancer may have no signs or symptoms. However, the following symptoms may occur:

- Constant coughing that becomes progressively worse or doesn't improve
- Shortness of breath

- Chest pain
- Wheezing
- Coughing up blood
- Continuous feeling of fatigue
- Unexplained and unintentional weight loss[6]

Treatment Options for Lung Cancer

Surgery may be an option for individuals who develop lung cancer, as is radiation. Chemotherapy is another treatment choice for people who are diagnosed with lung cancer. Researchers report that for individuals with non–small cell lung cancer at Stage I and II, most patients (about 69 percent) have surgery to remove the cancerous tumor, and about 25 percent of those who undergo surgery will also have radiation therapy. Among patients with Stage III or IV lung cancer, about half receive chemotherapy, either with or without radiation.[7] Targeted therapy medications are also increasingly used to treat advanced lung cancer.

Cervical Cancer

Cervical cancer is a cancer that forms in the cervix, which is an organ that connects the vagina and the uterus. It is a cancer that is more common among black women than women of other races and ethnicities. According to the American Cancer Society, an estimated 2,290 black women were diagnosed with cervical cancer in 2016, and the incidence rate (new cases) of cervical cancer is at least 41 percent higher in black women than in white women.[8] Another statistic also backs this up. In looking at the rate of cervical cancer among black women, cervical cancer occurred in 10.0 cases of every 100,000 black women in the 2008–2012 period, compared to the rate of 7.1 cases for white women.[9]

Cervical cancer is a preventable disease, and is often detected in a routine Pap smear performed by a gynecologist. This is an excellent reason to have an annual gynecological examination. Cervical cancer is very frequently associated with the presence of infection by the human papillomavirus (HPV) and this form of cancer can be prevented through screening, as can colorectal cancer.

Younger black women who are not yet sexually active can receive a vaccine for HPV from their doctors. The vaccine is given to females from about age 9 to age 26, according to the National Cancer Institute.[10]

Black women who have HPV and who also smoke have an elevated risk for cervical cancer, per the National Cancer Institute.[11]

BLACK WOMEN WITH CERVICAL CANCER IN MARYLAND RECEIVE LESS SURGERY THAN WHITE WOMEN

- Unfortunately, breast cancer is not the only type of cancer in which researchers have found racial disparities harmful to black women. Saroj Fleming and colleagues studied the treatments for both black women and white women in Maryland with cervical cancer over the period of 1992–2008. In this study, published in 2014, there were 1,301 white subjects and 733 black subjects. The researchers found that black women had 1.5 times the rate of receiving radiation therapy than white women and nearly the same rate (1.43) of receiving chemotherapy. However, black women were significantly less likely to receive brachytherapy than were white women, indicating a possible bias. In addition, black women had a much lower likelihood (0.51) of receiving surgery than white women. The black women were more likely to be diagnosed with later stages and metastatic cancers but the researchers adjusted the statistics to take this fact into account. The researchers concluded that black women with cervical cancer did not receive equivalent treatment to white women with this disease and that these differences contributed to racial disparities with the outcomes of women diagnosed with cervical cancer.

- They key problem may be lack of access. The researchers pointed out that gynecologic oncologists are available in limited areas and noted that in Prince George's County, Maryland, the incidence of cervical cancer was actually up to 25 percent lower than in other areas in the United States, yet the death rate was up to 25 percent higher in this county. They noted that there are a large number of black women in Prince George's County, but no gynecologic oncology services. Thus, black women in this area would need to travel to receive adequate treatment.[1]

- This is yet another example of racial disparities among black women with cancer in the United States, which needs to be addressed.

[1]Saroj Fleming et al., "Black and White Women in Maryland Receive Different Treatment for Cervical Cancer," *PLOS One* 9, no. 8 (August 2014), https://www.ncbi.nlm.nih .gov/pmc/articles/PMC4133178/pdf/pone.0104344.pdf (accessed October 12, 2016).

Signs and Symptoms of Cervical Cancer

Often there are no signs or symptoms of cervical cancer. However, some possible indicators of cervical cancer that should be checked out by your doctor are as follows:

- Bleeding between menstrual periods by women who are still menstruating
- Bleeding that occurs after douching, having sexual intercourse, or having a pelvic examination

- Having menstrual periods that last longer and are heavier than past periods
- Bleeding that occurs after a woman has experienced menopause
- Pain during sex
- Pelvic pain
- An increased vaginal discharge

Treatment Options for Cervical Cancer

Cervical cancer is treated by surgery, radiation, chemotherapy, and a combination of treatments, as are many forms of cancer. A gynecologic oncologist may treat this cancer, as may a general gynecologist, a radiation oncologist, and a medical oncologist.

Colorectal Cancer

There were 727,350 women of all races in the United States who were colorectal cancer survivors in 2016. These data include women who were just diagnosed with colorectal cancer as well as women who had this form of cancer many years ago. By 2026, it is estimated that there will be 885,940 survivors of colorectal cancer.[12]

Black women have a higher incidence rate of colorectal cancer than white women. The incidence of colorectal cancer in the period 2008–2012 was 44.1 women per 100,000 for black women and it was 36.2 for white women.[13] In addition, death rates from colorectal cancer are 41 percent higher among black women when compared to white women. This may be because of lower screening rates among black women, as well as differences in treatment and lower rates of recommended surgery and/or chemotherapy. However, the five-year survival rate for black women who were diagnosed with colorectal cancer has improved from 45 percent in the period 1975–1977 to the significantly better rate of 59 percent who survived this form of cancer in 2005–2011.[14]

Signs and Symptoms of Colorectal Cancer

There are usually few or no signs of colorectal cancer in the early stages. When symptoms do occur, they may include blood in the stools, abdominal pain, fatigue from anemia, a change in the shape of the stools from the usual shape for the person, and a feeling that the bowel has not completely emptied. The person may also have an unintentional weight loss. Some patients may present with acute abdominal pain resulting from a bowel blockage and requiring emergency surgery.

Treatment Options for Colorectal Cancer

The mainstay of therapy is radical surgery in patients with Stages I to III colon cancer. The large majority of those patients will have a partial colectomy, or removal of part of the colon. Chemotherapy for six months is always used after surgery in patients with Stage III disease and also in some patients with Stage II. Radiation therapy is used in rectal cancer only.[15]

Talking about Thyroid Cancer

Some experts believe that thyroid cancer may be more common among women who have had breast cancer. For example, in an analysis of research studies, researchers found that women who had breast cancer had a 1.55 greater risk for subsequently developing thyroid cancer. The researchers also found that women who had thyroid cancer *first* had an elevated risk for subsequently developing breast cancer. Possible reasons are shared hormonal risk factors, although further research is needed.[16] Some research presented at the Endocrine Society in 2015 indicates that radiation therapy for breast cancer may increase the risk for developing thyroid cancer.[17]

Thyroid cancer is one area where it is much more common among white women than black women. According to researchers, the incidence of thyroid cancer during the period 2008–2012 was 12.9 women per 100,000 black women, compared to 21.9 per 100,000 white women. The reasons for this racial disparity are unknown. Some people (like me) believe that the cause may be radiation therapy for breast cancer, but this is yet unproven.

In comments on the WebMD Internet site, some researchers have stated that the possible link between breast cancer and thyroid cancer may occur within five years of the breast cancer diagnosis. According to quotations from this article, researcher Jennifer Hong Kuo, said all breast cancer survivors should be checked for thyroid cancer within the first five years of their breast cancer diagnosis. She also advised at least one ultrasound scan of the thyroid gland.[18]

Signs and Symptoms of Thyroid Cancer

The person with thyroid cancer may have a lump in the neck that she can feel herself or that is detected by a physician. The individual may have trouble swallowing or even difficulty with breathing. There may also be pain in the neck or the throat that does not abate. If you have such symptoms, see your doctor, although most of the time they are not caused by thyroid cancer.

Treatment Options for Thyroid Cancer

Nearly all patients diagnosed with thyroid cancer have thyroid surgery and most are treated with a total thyroidectomy, or the removal of the entire thyroid gland. A partial thyroidectomy is another potential option, in which part of the thyroid is left behind. Some patients also receive radiation treatment after surgery. If the person has had a total thyroidectomy, then she will need to take thyroid replacement medication for the rest of her life. When the tumor cannot be totally removed, radiation therapy may follow surgery. Targeted drugs are used if the thyroid cancer has metastasized to other areas of the body.[19]

Important Preventive Tests That Check for Cancer

As mentioned earlier, preventive tests as well as an annual physical examination can help detect some forms of cancer, particularly cervical cancer and colorectal cancer. We've already discussed the importance of the mammogram in identifying possible breast cancer, so I won't repeat that information in this chapter. Just get an annual mammogram.

The Pap Smear

Invented by the Greek physiologist Georgios Papanicolaou in the 1940s, and widely accepted by the middle of the 20th century, the Pap smear is performed by a gynecologist who scrapes cells off the surface of the cervix and vagina to excise material to test for cancer or other diseases. Today many Pap smears are combined with tests for HPV, and the most common cause of cervical cancer in modern times.

Patients should not douche for 24 hours before having the Pap smear and they should also avoid having sex for 24 hours as well. The Pap smear should not be taken during menstruation because it can give an inaccurate reading of the test.[20]

The Colonoscopy

This examination will help the doctor discover if you have any precancerous polyps or other colonic problems that need to be treated. In most cases, polyps are removed during the procedure while the patient is under a light sedation. The problem of developing a potential cancer is averted because the polyps that could have become cancerous have been removed.

Preventive Actions against Cancer Recurrences (or First Time Occurrence) That You Can Take Now

Once you've had breast cancer, it's only common sense to have regular checkups and pay attention to your health. It's also a great idea to include plenty of vegetables and fruits in your diet because of their antioxidant (anti-cancer) value. If you still smoke after having had breast cancer, stop now. There are plenty of programs and some medications that can help you kick the habit. Last, increasing your level of physical activity and maintaining an ideal weight are both excellent ideas to help stave off the "Big C" of cancer from coming back into your life. Of course, no matter how much effort you put into your health, sometimes cancer does come back. In fact, younger black women who have had cancer (under age 50) have a greater risk for a recurrence with breast cancer than younger white women.[21]

Key preventive actions you can take to avoid cancer are the following:

- If you're overweight, lose weight.
- Eat more vegetables and fruits.
- Get hypertension under control.
- Cut back on alcohol consumption.
- Stop smoking.
- Increase exercising and movement.
- Consider the spiritual side.

If You're Overweight, Lose Weight

Many people have trouble losing weight because they feel they must lose a great deal of weight or they have failed. But if you are overweight or obese and lose even 10 pounds, it might mean the difference between type 2 diabetes and/or hypertension and the absence of these diseases. A greater weight loss would be even better. A weight loss will also likely make you less prone to developing some forms of cancer, such as colorectal cancer.

According to the National Cancer Institute, some studies have shown that black women have an elevated risk for gaining weight after their first experience with breast cancer. For example, some researchers have found

---

**BLACK BREAST CANCER SURVIVORS REALIZE THAT OVERWEIGHT
IS A PROBLEM WITH BREAST CANCER RECURRENCE**

- In a study of nearly 200 black female breast cancer survivors, research- ers asked the women what factors could increase their risk for a recur- rence of breast cancer. More than half (53 percent) said that overweight would increase the risk, and nearly half said that a lack of physical activity could also increase their risk for cancer recurrence. The researchers also looked at actual recurrences of breast cancer among these breast cancer survivors, and found that about 10 percent of the women with a body mass index of 25 or less developed breast cancer again, while 76 percent of the women with a higher body mass index have experienced a recurrence.[1]

- The women in this study realized that overweight and obesity increased the risk for a recurrence for breast cancer—and they were right. Doc- tors and other healthcare individuals should provide assistance and guidance to overweight breast cancer survivors who are interested in weight loss. Since research indicates that black women have a higher risk for a high body mass index than white women and they are at a risk for weight gain after a breast cancer diagnosis, it would be prudent to provide assistance on nutritional and weight loss assistance to this pop- ulation of women.

[1]Benjamin Ansa et al., "Beliefs and Behaviors about Breast Cancer Recurrence Risk Reduction among African American Breast Cancer Survivors," *International Journal of Environmental Research and Public Health* 13, no. 46 (2016), https://www.ncbi.nlm.nih .gov/pmc/articles/PMC4730437/ (accessed September 1, 2016).

---

that more than half of black female breast cancer survivors had gained weight after diagnosis, and they also gained more weight than their white or Asian counterparts. The black women gained an average of 13 pounds, compared to a weight gain of 6 pounds for the white woman and 1 pound for Asian women. The researchers noted that a weight gain increased the risk for a recurrence of breast cancer, as well as the development or wors- ening of type 2 diabetes and hypertension.[22]

Eat More Veggies and Fruit

Most doctors will advise their average patient to increase their consump- tion of fruits and vegetables, and this is particularly important if you are a breast cancer survivor. You can obtain valuable vitamins and antioxidants (cancer fighters) when you eat a steady diet of fruits and vegetables. The National Cancer Institute recommends 5–9 servings of vegetables and fruits per day.[23] You should also ask your doctor for any other recommended changes in your diet. Also, note that if you eat a healthy diet, you may find yourself losing some weight, which is also a positive step toward preventing future cancers. Also know that healthy eating will help protect you from cardiovascular diseases.

Get Hypertension under Control

If you have high blood pressure, as many black women do, it's important to get your hypertension under control. Some research indicates that hypertension alone may be a factor in the disparity of survival between black women and white women with breast cancer. For example, in a study of 416 black women and 838 white women in California, all of whom had breast cancer, the researchers followed up the subjects for nine years and found that the black women had a significantly lower survival rate. That is no surprise to readers of this book, because you have read many times that black women have a greater death risk from breast cancer than white women. However, here's some new information: The researchers found that hypertension contributed to an estimated 30 percent of the racial disparity between the black and white breast cancer survivors.[24] So high blood pressure was a big problem for the black women with breast cancer.

It's logical to assume that if you have high blood pressure, you may increase your survival prospects from breast cancer by getting your hypertension down to lower levels. Ask your doctor to help you. There are medications to treat high blood pressure, exercises, and also, of course, weight loss.

Cut Back on Alcohol Consumption

Excessive drinking can increase your risks for developing cancer again. Alcohol may seem to take your troubles away, but it really does not. On the other hand, mild alcohol consumption, such as a glass of wine per day, may be helpful for some women. Consult with your doctor for advice on alcohol consumption and whether it's acceptable or not.

Stop Smoking

It's very hard to give up a habit that you may have had for years and years, but if that habit is smoking and you've had breast cancer, smoking has got to go. Smoking is considered the single most preventable cause of many types of cancer, particularly lung cancer. There are nicotine replacement therapies as well as anti-smoking medications and even antidepressants that have been approved by the Food and Drug Administration as a means to stop smoking. Please, if you are a smoker, choose one of them and stop smoking as soon as possible!

Ask your doctor for help. Your physician may recommend a medication and/or a program for you to enter to help you quit smoking.

Increase Movement

Staying active is another good way to become healthier and make you less likely to develop a recurrence of breast cancer or the development of a new type of cancer. Exercise is also a good way to improve mood and decrease anxiety and depression. The mere act of moving about generates endorphins, which are brain chemicals that elevate a person's mood and make her feel better.

Consider the Spiritual Side

If you are a person who believes in God or a godlike entity, praying can really help when you have breast cancer, as well as later when the cancer treatment has ended. Having the Lord in my life and the faith that I have in Him has made this journey with cancer possible. Just knowing that the Lord was with me through every surgery, every treatment, and every procedure also helped me through this valley. Having faith and a good attitude was 100 percent of the cure for me mentally, which made it possible for me to fight this disease twice along with thyroid cancer. I personally believe that praying was extremely helpful for me also.

If you are not a religious person, you can learn to meditate or take classes in yoga to help you calm yourself and avoid the panic that can come surging to the forefront when you think about having cancer or maybe having a recurrence of cancer in the future. You may also gain considerable help from others, whether they are members of your religious group or members of a breast cancer support group.

Notes

1. American Cancer Society, *Cancer Facts & Figures for African Americans, 2016–2018*, Atlanta, GA, 2016.

2. Romano Demichell et al., "Racial Disparities in Breast Cancer Outcome: Insights into Host-Tumor Interactions," *Cancer* 110, no. 9 (November 1, 2007): 1880–1888.

3. Ibid.

4. Carol E. DeSantis et al., "Cancer Statistics for African Americans, 2016: Progress and Opportunities in Reducing Racial Disparities," *CA: A Cancer Journal for Clinicians* 66 (2016): 290–308.

5. American Cancer Society, "Tobacco and Cancer," January 2016, http://www.cancer.org/acs/groups/content/@nho/documents/document/tobaccoandcancerpdf.pdf (accessed October 2, 2016).

6. Centers for Disease Control and Prevention, "What Are the Symptoms of Lung Cancer," November 20, 2013, http://www.cdc.gov/cancer/lung/basic_info/symptoms.htm (accessed September 29, 2016).

7. Kimberly D Miller et al., "Cancer Treatment and Survivorship Statistics, 2016," *CA: A Cancer Journal for Clinicians* 66 (2016): 271–289.

8. American Cancer Society, *Cancer Facts & Figures for African Americans, 2016–2018*, Atlanta, GA, 2016.

9. Carol E. DeSantis et al., "Cancer Statistics for African Americans, 2016: Progress and Opportunities in Reducing Racial Disparities," *CA: A Cancer Journal for Clinicians* 66 (2016): 290–308.

10. Ibid.

11. National Cancer Institute, *What You Need to Know about Cervical Cancer*, Bethesda, MD, 2012.

12. Kimberly D. Miller et al., "Cancer Treatment and Survivorship Statistics, 2016," *CA: A Cancer Journal for Clinicians* 66 (2016): 271–289.

13. Carol E. DeSantis et al., "Cancer Statistics for African Americans, 2016: Progress and Opportunities in Reducing Racial Disparities," *CA: A Cancer Journal for Clinicians* 66 (2016): 290–308.

14. National Cancer Institute, *What You Need to Know about Cervical Cancer*, Bethesda, MD, 2012.

15. Ibid.

16. S. M. Nielsen et al., "The Breast-Thyroid Cancer Link: A Systematic Review and Meta-Analysis," *Cancer Epidemiology, Biomarkers & Prevention* 25, no. 2 (February 2016): 231–238.

17. *Science Daily*, "After Breast Cancer Diagnosis, Risk of Thyroid Cancer Goes Up," March 7, 2015, https://www.sciencedaily.com/releases/2015/03/150307095938.htm (accessed April 20, 2017).

18. Amy Norton, "Breast Cancer Health Center: Breast Cancer Survivors and Thyroid Cancer Risk," WebMD, 2015, http://www.webmd.com/breast-cancer/news/20150306/breast-cancer-survivors-may-have-higher-thyroid-cancer-risk (accessed October 10, 2016).

19. Ibid.

20. Irina Burd, "Pap Test," MedlinePlus, April 5, 2016, http://medlineplus,giv/ebct/article/003911.htm (accessed October 2, 2016).

21. Nicholas Diab et al., "Impact of Race and Tumor Subtype on Second Malignancy Risk in Women with Breast Cancer," *SpringerPlus* 5, no. 14 (2016).

22. Chanita Hughes Halbert, University of Pennsylvania, Philadelphia, "Weight Gain in African American Breast Cancer Survivors," Bethesda, MD: National Cancer Institute, Undated, http://cancercontrol.cancer.gov/ocs/resources/embracing-future/presentations/hughes-halbert.pdf (accessed September 27, 2016).

23. National Cancer Institute, *Facing Forward: Life after Cancer Treatment*, Bethesda, MD, May 2014, https://www.cancer.gov/publications/patient-educa tion/life-after-treatment.pdf (accessed October 1, 2016).

24. Dejana Braithwaite et al., "Hypertension Is an Independent Predictor of Survival Disparity between African-American and White Breast Cancer Patients," *International Journal of Cancer* 124 (2009): 1213–1219.

Cancer Is Gone: Be Happy— But Don't Let Your Guard Down

It's gone! The news is good, your doctor says the breast cancer is out of your body and you are joyful! Your body has emerged victorious in this very difficult struggle against cancer. In this chapter, I encourage you to relish your extreme happiness, while at the same time maintaining your vigilance against the cancer enemy. Cancer may be history for you, never recurring. But it's always best to be cautious because sadly cancer sometimes recurs or it may be diagnosed in another part of the body. In this chapter, I offer you cautionary advice to follow when you've had breast cancer before. I also discuss if and when the cancer comes back, whether it's another treatable case or it's an advanced cancer that cannot be cured.

Continue Regular Checkups

Your oncologist will tell you how often you will need to receive follow-up visits for your checkups. Follow-up care refers to the care that occurs after the treatment of breast cancer, such as physical examinations, imaging studies, laboratory tests, and other types of health care. Your doctor will determine the frequency of your medical encounters. However, for many people in the first three years after treatment for breast cancer, your doctor will want to see you every three to four months or thereabouts. Then for Years Four and Five after treatment, the doctor may wish to see you every 6–12 months. After the five-year point, the doctor likely will want you to have an annual checkup.[1]

When you have these medical follow-ups, the physician usually will go over your medical history, ask you specific questions about your health, and give you a physical examination. Be sure to volunteer information about any health problems you may be experiencing, such as pain, physical problems that impede your daily life or make it difficult to sleep at night, or issues such as fatigue and an unintended weight loss or gain. You may receive blood tests and imaging tests, such as CT scans or MRIs, based on symptoms.

Tell the doctor about *all* the medications that you take, including over-the-counter medications as well as herbal remedies, supplements, and vitamins. Many people think that only prescribed medicines "count," but the fact is that all drugs, including vitamins, herbs, and supplements or other non-prescribed medications, that you take represent data that are very important for the doctor to know about. Even aspirin can sometimes cause problems, such as blood thinning that can become a problem.

Coping with Chronic Fatigue

Researchers report that as many as a third of cancer survivors experience chronic fatigue up to six years after treatment.[2] Yet it's still important to push yourself to move about, go for walks, go bike riding, and perform at least minimal exercising. If you were active in the past before the onset of your breast cancer, you may not be able to achieve the same level of activity for a while, but keep moving! Regular exercise may help to protect you against a recurrence of cancer and also makes you feel good.

Dealing with Chronic Pain

Pain management may be a problem for some black women who are breast cancer survivors, whether it's pain stemming from cancer or pain caused by another medical problem, and there are some racial disparities regarding treatment for chronic pain. Doctors may worry about addiction to pain medication or side effects of pain drugs. In addition, the Centers for Disease Control released a new policy in 2016 that opposed the use of opioid narcotics for the use of chronic pain.[3] If you experience chronic pain subsequent to your breast cancer treatment, ask your doctor for suggestions to improve the condition. Non-narcotic medications may be available to assist you. For example, duloxetine (Cymbalta) is a noncontrolled medication that is also given to patients with chronic pain. Your doctor may also refer you to a pain specialist.

I strongly recommend regular exercise as a means to reduce pain because exercising releases endorphins, which are brain chemicals that can both improve mood and also decrease your pain levels.

Pay Attention to Certain Symptoms

If you experience any of the following symptoms, don't wait for the time of your checkup with your oncologist or primary care doctor. Instead, make an appointment to see her sooner to rule out any recurrence of breast cancer. These symptoms include the following:

- A lump in the breast or on the chest elsewhere
- A lump in the neck or in the pit of the arm
- A change in the shape of your breast
- A change in your skin color in the breast or the chest area
- A rash or swelling in the chest or the breast
- A sudden discharge from the nipple of the breast
- An unintended weight loss
- Vaginal bleeding that is abnormal (not menstruation)
- Shortness of breath or difficulty with breathing
- A cough that doesn't go away
- A new onset of back or hip pain

If you have any of the above symptoms or signs, be sure to tell your doctor right away so she can decide what, if anything, needs to be done.

Cope with Fears about Cancer Coming Back

After experiencing breast cancer and surviving it, many women still worry considerably that the cancer may come back. In fact, the National Cancer Institute says this is a common fear for people diagnosed with any form of cancer. They recommend these strategies:

- Educate yourself.
- Express your feelings, rather than burying them.
- Consider joining a support group.
- Don't blame yourself for having had cancer.
- Try to be positive.
- Realize you don't have to be constantly cheerful.

- Discover ways to relax.
- Stay active in activities that you enjoy.
- Identify areas where you do have control.

Educate Yourself

When you understand the basics of breast cancer, it helps to reduce the fear and anxiety that is often associated with the disease. It doesn't take it all away—cancer is scary, after all. But knowledge about the disease can significantly reduce the fear factor. Per the National Cancer Institute, people who are well informed about their illness experience a greater feeling of control than others.[4]

Express Your Feelings

A lot of people with cancer try to hide their feelings or bury them altogether, including their feelings of anger, fear, and sadness. Yet these are natural feelings that most people with cancer experience. Acknowledging and accepting that you have such emotions is a good step toward reducing future fears about a cancer recurrence. You may also wish to talk about how you feel to a spouse, a partner, or a friend.

Consider Joining a Support Group for Cancer Survivors

A support group is another opportunity to share feelings that others in the group can understand and relate to. There are many support groups for women with breast cancer, and you can meet with women in your area as well as on the Internet.

Before you decide to join a support group, check it out first, whether it's one that meets locally or on the web. Also, the National Cancer Institute recommends you ask yourself these questions regarding a support group:[5]

- Do I feel comfortable talking about personal issues? (Many groups can get very personal, which may be fine with you—or not.)
- Is the main purpose of the group to share tips or to talk about common feelings? Maybe you want some self-help information and are not so much interested in discussing emotions. On the other hand, feelings may be an area that you really want to explore.
- What do you hope to gain from joining the group? As in the previous question, you may wish to learn information you can't get elsewhere or you may just want to talk about feelings of anger, sadness, and other emotions. There are many groups and it's likely you can find one that will fulfill your needs.

Don't Blame Yourself

I've talked about risk factors for breast cancer in this book, such as obesity and smoking, but if you are an overweight smoker, the last thing you need to do is to overfocus on how your past behavior may have contributed to the diagnosis of breast cancer. Instead, realize that anyone can get cancer, including nonsmokers and thin people. It would be a very good idea to give up smoking and you may wish to lose some weight. But regard these actions as positive and healthy steps, rather than accentuating the negative—that they may have contributed to your breast cancer diagnosis.

Many people blame themselves when they initially are diagnosed with breast cancer and they continue to blame themselves well after treatment ends. This is a mistake.

It's also true that many people come up with silly reasons for why they may have developed breast cancer, such as that it's a punishment or karma for something that they have done wrong in the past—as if your cells had some sort of moral awareness separate from your brain. They don't.

Try to Be Positive

It's a good idea to work toward an overall positive attitude, which sometimes can be a sort of "Fake it until you make it." What this means is that if you are sad or depressed, but you often can find something amusing or funny, that can be a major mood-elevating experience. Avoid movies or televisions shows in which everyone dies and, instead, go for the comedies. In addition, focus on your wellness and try to maintain a healthy lifestyle. These types of actions will have a positive effect on you.

Realize You Don't Have to Be Constantly Cheerful

Although I've advised you to try to stay positive, this doesn't mean you need to paste a grin on your face 24/7/365. And other people should not expect you to act that way either. Some people who have had breast cancer or other forms of cancer say that they get sick of other people telling them to think positively. You have made it through to the other side of breast cancer, and that is a good thing. Sometimes you will feel angry or sad, and that is a natural part of life. You don't have to be constantly upbeat.

Discover Ways to Relax

Stress is a common problem for women who have had breast cancer, but there is a wide variety of ways to conquer stress. Progressive muscle relaxation is one way to alleviate stress, and yoga is another one.

The National Cancer Institute offers a stepwise exercise on progressive muscle relaxation, which follows.[6] Note that when you do the tensing part of the exercise, you should tighten your muscles in the part of your body where you are concentrating as much as you can. Then when you relax, send all the tension out of your body until it's completely gone.

1. Find a quiet place where you can rest alone for at least 20 minutes. Tell other people that you need some alone time now.

2. Ensure that the setting really is a relaxed one. You may wish to dim the lights or close the blinds. You can lie down or sit in a comfortable chair such as a recliner.

3. Find a comfortable position and then close your eyes. Clear your mind of all distractions.

4. Take deep and calming breaths, breathing slowly and deeply. Your stomach should go up and down with each breath.

5. Starting at one part of your body, you will tense, hold, and then completely relax your muscles in that part of the body. If one part of your body feels painful when you tense up, then stop the tensing and just go with the relaxation part of the exercise.

6. Completely release all the tension in your muscles. One after the other, tense, hold the tension, and then completely relax your:

   - right and left arms. Make a tight fist and feel the tension all the way up to your shoulder. Then release it all, letting the tension totally flow out of your body.

   - lips, eyes, and forehead. Raise your eyebrows high, pucker up your lips, and then grin widely so you look like a fool. (Remember, if you followed my advice, there's no one there to criticize you.) Then relax all the tension out.

   - jaws and neck: Stick your jaw out as far as you can, hold it, and then relax so much so that your chin drops down to your chest.

   - shoulders: Shrug your shoulders up high and toward your neck, hold this position, and then relax it all out.

   - stomach: Suck in your stomach as if there were an invisible corset tightening you up. Hold it, and then let it all out.

- lower back: Arch your lower back gently, with your stomach sticking out. Do this part of the exercise gently since lower back muscles are often very tense. Then feel the tension flow out of your lower back.

- buttocks: Squeeze your butt tightly, hold it, and then let it all out.

- feet: Point your feet downward like a ballet dancer, and then relax completely.

7. See how your different body parts feel, and if there's still any tension anywhere, such as in your low back, neck, or anywhere else, repeat the exercise in these areas of your body.

Stay Active in Activities That You Enjoy

You probably gave up a lot of your favorite activities during your cancer treatment. After treatment ends, it's time to get back to your favorite hobbies and other activities. Rather than staying in your house fixating about whether you might get cancer again, get out of the house and engage in activities that you enjoy, whether it's getting together with your friends, jogging, engaging in church activities, or engaging in other positive actions that involve at least some movement.

Identify Areas Where You *Do* Have Control

Many people say that having cancer feels like a complete loss of control to them. Of course, even without cancer, you can never have total control of your life, but there are some areas that you can take charge of, even with breast cancer, and identifying them and acting upon them is a positive and helpful action. For example, making lifestyle changes such as quitting smoking or losing weight are positive personal choices that you can choose to make to control your life. Creating your own daily schedule is another area of life where you can exercise your own control.

If and When Breast Cancer Comes Back: Initial Reactions

It is possible for breast cancer to come back. I have had breast cancer twice, and consequently, I am a survivor of both of these cancers. I also developed thyroid cancer, a disease which I discussed in Chapter Nine. So, how do you feel if you get another cancer diagnosis? Pretty awful. It's not as shocking as the first time, but I don't want to downplay the anger, grief, and fear that happens with a second-time diagnosis of cancer. You may also feel like, how could this have happened to you again, after you

---

LOW VITAMIN D LEVELS LINKED TO BREAST CANCER

As part of prevention against a recurrence of breast cancer, it's a good idea to have your doctor periodically check your vitamin D blood levels. Researchers have found that many black women have low levels of vitamin D. In a study of nearly 3,000 black women who had been diagnosed with breast cancer in the United States, researchers found that 22 percent were vitamin D deficient and 25 percent had insufficient blood levels of vitamin D. The researchers also found that black women in the lowest quarter of vitamin D levels had a 23 percent elevated risk for breast cancer compared to those black women with high levels. They noted that preventing vitamin D deficiency may be one means to reduce the risk for breast cancer.[1]

This is good information to also share with your friends, to help them prevent against getting breast cancer! They can ask their doctors to test their blood levels of vitamin D. Low blood levels can be corrected with taking prescribed vitamin D. (Do not assume that you are deficient in vitamin D because you are black. Get a test to determine your levels first. No one should take medications that are not needed.)

[1]Julie R. Palmer et al., "Predicted 25-Hydroxyvitamin D in Relation to Incidence of Breast Cancer in a Large Cohort of African American Women," *Breast Cancer Research* 18, no. 86 (2016), https://breast-cancer-research.biomedcentral.com/articles/10.1186/s13058-016-0745-x (accessed October 12, 2016).

---

did everything the doctor said to do the first time and with his help, you beat cancer before. It doesn't seem fair. And it isn't fair. I could say here that life isn't always "fair," but a second-time cancer diagnosis seems especially unjust. However, you work your way through all these negative feelings and then you move on, doing everything you can to help your oncologist to help you overcome the cancer.

When the Cancer Is Curable

If breast cancer comes back, it often is a curable type. You'll go through pretty much the same drill to diagnose the cancer as you went through the first time around, such as having a biopsy, imaging scans, and other tests that are taken as your doctor recommends. Your cancer will also be staged to determine the best treatments.

My second bout of breast cancer was diagnosed at Stage IIA. It occurred in the same breast as where I had been diagnosed with breast cancer for the first time, but this time, I decided to get a double mastectomy, because I wasn't taking any chances for my second bout with breast cancer. And I am very glad that I made that choice, because a subsequent check of the tissue from my other breast later revealed that cancer was lurking there too! You may need surgery, radiation, chemotherapy, and other treatments that your doctor recommends, and that have been discussed in this book.

When the Cancer Has Spread and Prolonging of Life Is the Plan

Sometimes when breast cancer recurs, it could have spread to other parts of the body. Of course, sometimes when a person is diagnosed with breast cancer for the first time, she may have metastatic cancer. And it is also possible that the second cancer diagnosis could be an advanced cancer that cannot be cured.

If the cancer has spread, then treatment is given to prolong life and decrease symptoms. If you have metastatic breast cancer, your oncologist has a variety of cancer-fighting weapons in his arsenal. Chemotherapy is one option, and hormone therapy is another one to consider. In some limited cases, doctors may choose surgery or radiation therapy to treat the metastatic breast cancer.

Thinking about End-of-Life Issues

Every person dies but people with metastatic cancer know that their life span will end sooner than they would have liked. Yet there are still some areas where you can exercise control and ease the suffering of your loved ones. For example, you can consider the following issues and the decisions associated with them:

- Deciding for or against continued treatment
- Deciding for or against a "Do Not Resuscitate" order
- Creating a living will
- Designating a medical surrogate
- Other end-of-life decisions

Deciding for or against Continued Treatments with Machines

The person with advanced cancer needs to make difficult decisions well before she is confronted with these choices. For example, if you can no longer eat food, are you willing to be fed with a nasogastric tube? If you should develop difficulty with breathing, would you be willing to receive oxygen through a mask or a tube—or a ventilator that breathes for you? And if your kidneys fail, will you be willing to undergo kidney dialysis, in which a machine cleanses your blood of impurities, since your kidneys can no longer handle that task? These are issues that you can state in a living will.

Deciding for or against a "Do Not Resuscitate" Order

Another major health-related issue is whether you favor or oppose a "do not resuscitate" (DNR) order, which means that if your heart stops working, do you wish to receive cardiopulmonary resuscitation (CPR)? Or not? These are very tough decisions to make, but it's better that you make them yourself than to let your relatives guess at what you would really want in such a situation. Experts say that the DNR is one of the most commonly known medical abbreviations today, although the term was first used in the 1970s. Before then, patient charts used an array of symbols or "codes" to denote a patient who should not be resuscitated. Then in 1974, the American Medical Association recommended a formal documentation of this decision in the patient's medical record. Some doctors have stated that a better term would be "DNAR" or "do not attempt resuscitation," as when the patient is extremely unlikely to live much beyond a CPR attempt.[7]

Creating a Living Will

A living will is a document that covers the kind of healthcare decisions that you want taken in your own case, in the event that you become so ill that you can't tell others what you want. The information already discussed, such as the DNR and whether you wish machines to help maintain your life, as well as other choices are included in a living will. The living will also often covers situations such as tissue or organ donation, whether you would want dialysis in the event your kidneys failed, whether you wish to have a DNR set in place, and other situations.

Each state has its own laws on how a living will should be accomplished. You can contact a family law attorney for assistance or some individuals create their own living wills after checking state laws.

Designating a Healthcare Agent/Medical Surrogate/ Medical Power of Attorney

Many people with advanced cancer choose a family member or friend to make medical decisions for them in the event they can no longer make such decisions themselves. Be sure to tell your healthcare agent what types of health care you support and don't support—and also put this information in writing in a living will.

Other End-of-Life Decisions

You may wish to create a will that designates the people who should receive your share of your home and any other assets that you possess. If you are a single parent, it's also a good idea to determine whom you want to raise your children in the event of your death, and make sure that this person or people are willing to take over parenting for you before you list this information in your will. Give them a copy of the will too.

Notes

1. California Department of Health Services, Cancer Detection and Treatment Branch, *A Woman's Guide to Breast Cancer Treatment*, Sacramento, CA, January 2016; National Cancer Institute, *Facing Forward: Life after Cancer Treatment*, Bethesda, MD, May 2014.

2. J. M. Jones et al., "Cancer-Related Fatigue and Associated Disability in Post-Treatment Cancer Survivors," *Journal of Cancer Survivors* 10, no. 1 (February 2016): 51–61.

3. L. D. Dowell, T. M. Haegerich, and R. Chou, "CDC Guideline for Prescribing Opioids for Chronic Pain—United States, 2016," *Morbidity and Mortality Weekly Report* 2016; 65 (No. RR-1): 1–49, http://dx.doi.org/10.15585/mmwr.rr6501e1 (accessed October 12, 2016).

4. Ibid.

5. National Cancer Institute, *Facing Forward: Life after Cancer Treatment*, Bethesda, MD, May 2014.

6. Ibid.

7. Jeffrey P. Burns, and Robert D. Truong, "The DNR Order after 40 Years," *New England Journal of Medicine* (August 11, 2016): 504–506.

Conclusion

I believe that knowledge is power, and that is a key reason why I wrote this book. My goal is to empower black women who have breast cancer, as well as to help their friends and families, and to do so by providing the information that you need on this disease. Breast cancer is not a taboo subject anymore. It is a real disease and we can talk about it with our family and friends. We don't have to go through this experience alone without being armed with knowledge and power. Now we have come to the end of my book and this is my opportunity to summarize the key points I've tried to convey to you. There is a great deal of research on breast cancer and black women, and I have tried to identify and read as much of it as possible. This was sometimes a discouraging task, because so often I found disheartening results in the disparities of the treatment and outcomes for black women with breast cancer when they were compared to white women or women of other races. Most researchers don't know why these disparities exist, although they have many hypotheses to try to explain them.

Does this mean that this is a very bad time to be a black woman with breast cancer? My attitude is that when you shine light on a problem, it brings increased awareness and concern about that problem. This was one of my goals in writing this book: to educate black women about breast cancer and also to reveal the very real problems that black women with breast cancer face today, so that hopefully in the near future, the root causes of these problems can be identified and resolved.

I also think it's important to consider the issue of racial disparities between black women and white women with regard to breast cancer. I think I have made a strong case, based on a review of a great deal of research that such disparities clearly exist. As to *why* they exist, no one knows for sure. It could be poverty, although some research indicates that affluent black women have worse outcomes in terms of their five-year survival than rich white women.[1] So maybe it's genetics that's the key issue. The key problem could also be lack of access to good health care. Or it could be such issues as a high level of obesity among black women— or maybe it's fear of doctors. There may be several key issues that are contributing to racial disparities in treatment of breast cancer in black women. There may also be as-yet unidentified factors that are driving this problem. And let's face it, the issue could also be an underlying racism that still permeates our society. Maybe it's 10 percent of the cause of the racial disparity or maybe it's as low as 1–2 percent. But it's likely there, and our society needs to move beyond it so that black women receive treatment for their breast cancer that's just as good as the treatment received by white women.

What can a black woman with breast cancer do to ensure that she receives the best possible treatment? One way is to read this book and to understand the different types of breast cancer, how they are diagnosed, and what their treatment options are. I also strongly encourage you to ask your doctor questions. In addition, if a physician steers you toward a particular treatment, what are her reasons? If you break down what the doctor is telling you, does it seem to make sense? If not, ask more questions. If the suggested treatment still seems "off" to you, then get a second opinion. The first doctor could be completely right or she could be totally wrong. But this is your body and your life, and it's important to stand up for yourself.

There are also ways to increase your survival rate from breast cancer after treatment, and research clearly shows that ending a smoking habit, ridding yourself of excess weight, and getting control of hypertension are all good ways to decrease your risk for a cancer recurrence. Of course, no matter what you do, sometimes it just happens anyway and the cancer occurs for the first time or a second time. That means you could be a non-smoker, weigh 100 pounds, have fabulous blood pressure, and never drink. And yet you get breast cancer anyway. You are what researchers call an "outlier," or an unusual person, but it happens. In that case, work with your doctors, keep stress under control as best you can, and follow the course your doctor lays out for you.

Many women find that spirituality and a relationship with God or a higher power helps them get through the terrible psychological strain of breast cancer, while others find that calming exercises or yoga help them manage their emotions and feelings. Don't bottle them up—or they'll burst out like a can of carbonated soda that someone shook up. Find a support group to help you and talk to other women with breast cancer.

I hope I have helped you in your battle against breast cancer, and that you are ready and willing to fight against this terrible disease.

Note

1. S. Lehrer, S. Green, and K. E. Rosenzweig, "Affluence and Breast Cancer," *Breast Journal* 22, no. 5 (September 2016): 564–567.

Organizations That Can Help

National Breast and Cervical Cancer Early Detection Program (NBC-CEDP) helps poor and uninsured women obtain clinical breast examinations and mammograms. It's available in every state (https://nccd.cdc.gov/dcpc_Programs/index.aspx#/1).

Black Women with Breast Cancer

African American Breast Cancer Alliance
http://aabcainc.org/

Black Women's Health Imperative
http://www.blackwomenshealth.org

Celebrating Life Foundation
http://www.celebratinglife.org/

Living beyond Breast Cancer group
http://www.lbbc.org/african-american

Sisters Network
www.sistersnetworkinc.org

Other Websites with Helpful Information

American Cancer Society
http://www.cancer.org

American Society of Plastic and Reconstructive Surgeons
http://www.plasticsurgery.org

CancerCare
http://www.cancercare.org

Cancer Research and Prevention Foundation
http://www.preventcancer.org

Cancer Survivors Network blog (on American Cancer Society site)
http://csn.cancer.org/forum/127?_ga=1.88529179.1454366601.1456944508

Centers for Disease Control and Prevention
www.cdc.gov

National Cancer Institute
http://www.cancer.gov

National Cancer Institute Designated Cancer Centers
http://www.cancer.net/navigating-cancer-care/cancer-basics/cancer-care-team/
   find-nci-designated-cancer-center

National Coalition for Cancer Survivorship
http://www.canceradvocacyh.org

Physician Data Query
http://www.cancer.gov/publications/pdq

Susan G. Komen for the Cure
http://ww5.komen.org/

Glossary

Anti-estrogen therapy
Treatment that blocks the action of estrogen.

Aromatase inhibitors (AIs)
A special category of hormone medications used to treat breast cancer in some women.

Biopsy
A special test to determine whether cancer is present or not by extracting tissue from the tumor. A pathologist analyzes the sample to determine if the tumor is cancerous as well as how advanced the cancer is.

Brachytherapy
Radiation that is administered inside the body as a treatment against breast cancer or other forms of cancer.

BRCA and BRCA2
Refers to Breast Cancer A and Breast Cancer B, two genes that increase the risk for breast cancer.

Breast cancer
A malignant tumor that originates in the breast.

Breast cancer survivor
Person who is still alive despite having had breast cancer. There are nearly 3 million breast cancer survivors in the United States.

Breast implants
Silicone or saline pockets that are surgically implanted into the breast at some point after a mastectomy. Some women who have never had breast cancer obtain breast implants to make their breasts larger. Some women who have had mastectomies do not choose to have breast implants.

Breast-sparing surgery
Refers to partial surgical removal of the breast. Also known as lumpectomy, breast-conserving surgery, or quadrectectomy. The person may receive breast implants at some point after this surgery or may choose to not have implants.

Cervical cancer
A cancer that forms in the cervix, which is an organ that connects the vagina and the uterus. It is often detected in a routine Pap smear performed by a gynecologist. Cervical cancer is frequently associated with the presence of infection by the human papillomavirus (HPV). This form of cancer is more common in black women than in white women.

Chemobrain
Slang term for the confusion and forgetfulness that may accompany chemotherapy treatment.

Chemoradiation
Treatment for cancer that includes both chemotherapy and radiation therapy. It is also sometimes called chemoradiotherapy.

Chemotherapy
Refers to special medications that are administered to either kill the cancer cells directly or prevent them from continuing to divide and multiply. These treatments may be administered orally, by injection, or intravenously. In some cases, chemotherapy is topically administered.

Clinical study
A research study that is performed to test a medication or other treatment on humans. Studies may test new methods of screening, diagnosis, and treatment, or on the prevention of breast cancer or other forms of cancer.

Colorectal cancer
A common form of cancer that affects the colon or rectum. Blacks have a higher risk for colorectal cancer than whites.

Computerized tomography scan
An imaging study that uses a computer that is linked to an X-ray machine, and this device allows the physician to obtain a picture of the abdomen and chest to check for cancer. Sometimes contrast material is given orally or by injection to highlight areas of the body. The CT scan may also be used to check if the breast cancer has spread to the liver or lungs, both common sites where breast cancer spreads. Also known as a CT scan, CAT scan, computed tomography scan, and computerized axial tomography scan.

Ductal carcinoma
A type of cancer that originates in the tubes (the ducts) of the breast that send milk to the nipple if a woman breastfeeds a baby.

Endocrine therapy
Another term that refers to anti-estrogen therapy to treat cancer.

Follow-up care
Care that occurs subsequent to the treatment of breast cancer, such as physical examinations, imaging studies, laboratory tests, and other types of care.

Genetic testing
Blood or saliva testing to determine if a woman has genetic mutations that increase her risk for the rapid growth of breast cancer.

Hair prosthesis
A wig that may be used by a woman who has lost her hair due to chemotherapy. Insurance companies may use the term "hair prosthesis."

HER2 positive
Refers to the human epidermal genetic factor 2 protein, a specific protein that can cause breast cancer to grow faster. Some individuals are HER2 negative. Knowing the HER2 status of a woman's breast cancer helps the doctor to determine the best treatment to use.

Hormone blockers
Medications that block female hormones such as estrogen in the treatment of breast cancer.

Implant radiation therapy
A form of radiation therapy in which radioactive material is inserted through catheters or other means directly into or near a cancerous tumor. Also known as brachytherapy or radiation brachytherapy.

Inflammatory breast cancer
A type of breast cancer that is dangerous and rapidly growing. It causes warmness and skin irritation because the cancer cells block the lymph vessels in the skin. Black women have a greater risk for inflammatory breast cancer than other women.

Intensity-modulated radiation therapy (IMRT)
A very targeted form of radiation therapy that uses computers to generate radiation from many different angles directly at the cancerous tumor. This type of therapy preserves healthy tissue that is nearby the tumor.

Interstitial brachytherapy
One of the two primary types of brachytherapy. Radioactive material is placed into one or two tiny tubes/catheters that are then inserted through a small incision in the breast.

Intracavity brachytherapy
A type of procedure in which a special device is inserted directly into the breast through a tiny catheter. The inserted end is then expanded so it can remain in

place during treatment. Tiny irradiated pellets are sent to the breast through this catheter and left in place for a short period.

Intraoperative radiation therapy
Radiation therapy that is administered within the same time frame as surgery.

Invasive breast cancer
Breast cancer that has spread beyond the point where it originally developed.

Linear accelerator
A device that administers external radiation therapy to women with breast cancer.

Lobular carcinoma
A malignant tumor that originates in 1 of about 20 lobes located in the breast.

Local cancer
Also known as localized cancer. Refers to cancer that has not grown far beyond the original site.

Localized therapy
Treatment that concentrates on the area where the cancer originates, such as surgery or radiation therapy.

Luminal A breast cancer
A genetic type of breast cancer that is common, although more common in white women with breast cancer than black women. The prognosis is often good with this form of cancer.

Luminal B breast cancer
Another genetic type of cancer and one with a less favorable prognosis than with Luminal A breast cancer.

Lumpectomy
Surgery that removes the cancerous area of the breast and the tissue around. Also known as breast-conserving surgery.

Lung cancer
The most common form of cancer. It originates in the lungs and is often caused by smoking. The two primary forms of lung cancer are small cell lung cancer and non–small cell lung cancer. The type is diagnosed based on the appearance of the cells under a microscope.

Lymphadenectomy
A surgical procedure that involves the removal of lymph nodes and the checking of a sample of removed tissue under a microscope for the presence of cancer.

Lymphedema
A swelling of the lymph glands that may be painful. It may be caused by damaged or blocked lymph vessels or by their removal during surgery.

Lymph node
Small bean-like structure that is an important part of the immune system of the body. Hundreds of lymph glands are located throughout the body and they are connected by lymph vessels. There are up to 40 lymph glands in the underarm area (axilla). Also known as a lymph gland.

Magnetic resonance imaging (MRI)
A procedure in which a computer that is connected to a powerful magnet creates very detailed pictures of the inside of the body. The MRI differentiates healthy tissue from diseased tissue. Also known as nuclear magnetic resonance imaging.

Mammogram
A special imaging study used to detect breast cancer. A screening mammogram is used if there is no suspicion of cancer, while a diagnostic mammogram, a more detailed study, is used if the radiologist believes that breast cancer may be present.

Metastasis
Cancer that has spread beyond its original site. The cancer cells break off from the original tumor and travel through the lymph system or the bloodstream to form a new tumor elsewhere in the body. This tumor has the same cells as the original tumor, so if breast cancer cells lodge in the lung, they are still breast cancer cells, rather than lung cancer cells.

Monoclonal antibodies
Medications that were developed to target an immune system protein that helps breast cancer grow.

Myths
Commonly held beliefs that are not true. For example, some women believe that surgery causes cancer to spread, which it does not. There are many myths about breast cancer in particular as well as cancer in general.

National Cancer Institute
Organization that is part of the National Institutes of Health of the federal Department of Health and Human Services. The National Cancer Institute funds, coordinates, and conducts research on cancer as well as providing training and information on the cause, diagnosis, prevention, and treatment of cancer.

Oncologist
Medical doctor who specializes in the treatment of cancer. A radiation oncologist specializes in treatment using radiation therapy while a medical oncologist uses chemotherapy or hormone therapy to treat cancer. A surgeon who treats cancer with surgery may be called an oncologic surgeon or simply a surgeon.

Pathologist
Medical doctor who analyzes the results of removed tissue to determine if cancer is present.

Radiation therapy
Use of radiation to destroy breast cancer or other forms of cancer. The two primarily forms of radiation therapy used in breast cancer are external beam radiation therapy (EBRT) and brachytherapy.

Reconstructive surgery
Surgery performed by a plastic surgeon to create the natural appearance of the breast subsequent to a mastectomy.

Risk factors
Indicators that increase the probability that a person may develop breast cancer, such as a family history of breast cancer, obesity, smoking, being black, and other risk factors.

Secondary tumor
When breast cancer from one part of the body migrates elsewhere, this is referred to as a secondary tumor. It is still breast cancer, although not located in the breast.

Sentinel lymph node biopsy
A procedure in which a radioactive substance and/or a blue dye is injected by the surgeon near the tumor. The substance will go to one or more lymph nodes first, and it is these nodes that are removed by the surgeon to check for cancer.

Staging
The process by which the physician predicts how fast a tumor is growing and what its current level of severity is. Staging helps the doctor determine how to treat the breast cancer. Staging is performed with a biopsy as well as with imaging studies such as a CT scan.

Support group
Local, regional, or Internet organization that provides emotional support and information. There are many support groups for women with breast cancer.

Systemic therapy
Treatment that includes the entire body, such as chemotherapy or hormone therapy.

Targeted therapy
Therapy that uses drugs or other substances to attack certain types of cancer cells, such as sells that are HER2 positive.

Thyroid cancer
Cancer that occurs in the thyroid gland, located in the neck.

Thyroid guard
A special shield that covers and protects the thyroid gland during radiation treatments or X-rays of any type, including dental X-rays.

TNM staging
A type of staging in which the person's tumor is classified with regard to three items, including the tumor size (the "T" in TNM), the lymph node status (the "N" in TNM), and last, whether the cancer has metastasized or spread or it has not (the "M" in TNM).

Triple-negative breast cancer
A type of cancer that has neither estrogen or progesterone hormonal receptors nor the presence of the HER2-positive protein. This form of breast cancer grows rapidly and does not respond to hormone therapy. Black women have a high risk for triple-negative breast cancer, although women of any race or ethnicity may develop this form of cancer.

Bibliography

Ademuywa, Foluso D., et al. "United States Breast Cancer Mortality Trends in Young Women According to Race." *Cancer* 121, no. 9 (2015): 1469–1476.

Agency for Healthcare Research and Quality. *Having a Breast Biopsy: A Guide for Women and Their Families.* Agency for Healthcare Research and Quality. Rockville, MD: Agency for Healthcare Research and Quality, April 2010. https://hvc.acponline.org/AHRQ/Breast_Biopsy.pdf (accessed May 6, 2016).

Akinyemiju, Tomi, Swati Sakhuja, and Neomi Vin-Raviv. "Racial and Socio-Economic Disparities in Breast Cancer Hospitalization Outcomes by Insurance Status." *Cancer Epidemiology* 43 (2016): 63–69.

American Cancer Society. *Breast Cancer.* Atlanta, GA: American Cancer Society, May 4, 2016. http://www.cancer.org/acs/groups/cid/documents/webcon tent/003090-pdf.pdf (accessed September 10, 2016).

American Cancer Society. *Cancer Facts & Figures for African Americans: 2016–2018.* Atlanta, GA: American Cancer Society, 2016. http://www.cancer.org/acs/groups/content/@editorial/documents/document/acspc-047403.pdf (accessed October 18, 2016).

American Cancer Society. *A Guide to Radiation Therapy.* Atlanta, GA: American Cancer Society, June 30, 2015.

American Cancer Society. "Lobular Carcinoma in Situ (LCIS)."April 21, 2016. http://www.cancer.org/healthy/findcancerearly/womenshealth/non-can cerousbreastconditions/non-cancerous-breast-conditions-lobular-carci noma-in-situ (accessed September 24, 2016).

American Cancer Society. "Radiation Therapy for Breast Cancer." September 13, 2016. http://www.cancer.org/cancer/breastcancer/detailedguide/breast-can cer-treating-radiation (accessed September 18, 2016).

American Psychiatric Association. *Diagnostic and Statistical Manual of Mental Disorders (Fifth Edition) (DSM-5).* Washington, DC: American Psychiatric Association, 2013.

Amirikia, Kathryn C., Paul Mills, Jason Bush, and Lisa A. Newman. "Higher Population-Based Incidence Rates of Triple-Negative Breast Cancer among Young African-American Women." *Cancer* 117, no. 12 (June 15, 2011): 2747–2753.

Andic, Fundagul, et al. "Treatment Adherence and Outcome in Women with Inflammatory Breast Cancer: Does Race Matter?" *Cancer* (December 15, 2011): 5485–5492.

Ansa, Benjamin, et al. "Beliefs and Behaviors about Breast Cancer Recurrence Risk Reduction among African American Breast Cancer Survivors." *International Journal of Environmental Research and Public Health* 13, no. 46 (2016). https://www.ncbi.nlm.nih.gov/pmc/articles/PMC4730437/ (accessed April 7, 2017).

Baan, Robert, et al. "Carcinogenicity of Alcoholic Beverages." *Lancet Oncology* 8, no. 4 (April 2007): 292–293. http://www.thelancet.com/pdfs/journals/lanonc/PIIS1470-2045(07)70099-2.pdf (accessed September 23, 2016).

Balasubramanian, Bijal A., et al. "Black Medicaid Beneficiaries Experience Breast Cancer Treatment Delays More Frequently than Whites." *Ethnicity & Disease* 22 (Summer 2012): 288–294.

Beck, Melinda. "Alternative Way to Treat Early-Stage Breast Cancer with Radiation." *Wall Street Journal,* August 24, 2015. http://www.wsj.com/articles/alternative-way-to-treat-early-stage-breast-cancer-with-radiation-1440448587 (accessed September 15, 2016).

Bodai, Balazs I., and Philip Tuso. "Breast Cancer Survivorship: A Comprehensive Review of Long-Term Medical Issues and Lifestyle Recommendations." *The Permanente Journal* 19, no. 2 (Spring 2015): 48–75.

Boyle, P. "Triple-Negative Breast Cancer: Epidemiological Considerations and Recommendations." *Annals of Oncology* 23, Supp. 6 (2012): v7–v12.

Bradley, Patricia K. "African American Women and Breast Cancer Issues." In *African American Women's Life Issues Today: Vital Health and Social Matters*, edited by Catherine Fisher Collins, 63–83. Santa Barbara, CA: Praeger, 2013.

Braithwaite, Dejana, et al. "Hypertension Is an Independent Predictor of Survival Disparity between African-American and White Breast Cancer Patients." *International Journal of Cancer* 124 (2009): 1213–1219.

Breslin, Tara M., and Sandra A. Finestone. "What Patients Need to Know about Breast Biopsies." Medscape. http://www.medscape.org/viewarticle/567831_print (accessed May 10, 2016).

Burd, Irina. "Pap Test." MedlinePlus, April 5, 2016. http://medlineplus,giv/ebct/article/003911.htm (accessed October 2, 2016).

Burns, Jeffrey P., and Robert D. Truong. "The DNR Order after 40 Years." *New England Journal of Medicine* (August 11, 2016): 504–506.

California Department of Health Services, Cancer Detection and Treatment Branch. *A Woman's Guide to Breast Cancer Treatment.* Sacramento, CA: California Department of Health Services, Cancer Detection and Treatment Branch, January 2016. http://www.mbc.ca.gov/Publications/Brochures/breast_cancer_english.pdf (accessed October 17, 2016).

Centers for Disease Control and Prevention. "What Are the Symptoms of Breast Cancer?" http://www.cdc.gov/cancer/breast/basic_info/symptoms.htm (accessed May 5, 2016).

Chartier, Karen G., Patrice A. C. Vaeth, and Raul Caetano. "Focus on Ethnicity and the Social and Health Harms from Drinking." *Alcohol Research: Current Reviews* 35, no. 2 (2013): 229–237.

Dab, Nicholas, et al. "Impact of Race and Tumor Subtypes on Second Malignancy Risk in Women with Breast Cancer." *Springer Plus* 5, no. 14 (2016). https://www.ncbi.nlm.nih.gov/pmc/articles/PMC4703603/pdf/40064_2015_Article_1657.pdf (accessed April 7, 2017).

Daher, M. "Cultural Beliefs and Values in Cancer Patients." *Annals of Oncology* 22, Supp. 3 (2012): iii66–iii69.

D'Arcy, Monica, et al. "Race-Associated Biological Differences among Luminal A Breast Tumors." *Breast Cancer Research and Treatment* 152, no. 2 (2015): 437–448.

Demichell, Romano, et al. "Racial Disparities in Breast Cancer Outcome: Insights into Host-Tumor Interactions." *Cancer* 110, no. 9 (November 1, 2007): 1880–1888.

Der, Edmund M., et al. "Triple-Negative Breast Cancer in Ghanaian women: The Karle Bu Teaching Hospital Experience." *The Breast Journal* (2015): 627–633. doi:10.1111/tbj.12527.

DeSantis, Carol E., et al. "Breast Cancer Statistics, 2015: Convergence of Incidence Rates between Black and White Women." *CA: A Cancer Journal for Clinicians* 66, no. 1 (January/February 2016): 31–42.

DeSantis, Carol E., et al. "Cancer Statistics for African Americans, 2016: Progress and Opportunities in Reducing Racial Disparities." *CA: A Cancer Journal for Clinicians* 66, no. 4(July–August 2016): 290–308.

Di Leo, A., et al. "Optimizing Treatment in Luminal Breast Cancer. Introduction: Luminal A and B: How Curable Are They?" *Annals of Oncology* 23, Supp. 9 (2012). http://annonc.oxfordjournals.org/content/23/suppl_9/ix27.full (accessed October 12, 2016).

Dowell, L. D., T. M. Haegerich, and R. Chou. CDC Guideline for Prescribing Opioids for Chronic Pain—United States, 2016. *Morbidity and Mortality Weekly Report Recomm Rep* 2016; 65 (No. RR-1): 1–49.

Enewold, Lindsey, et al. "Breast Reconstruction after Mastectomy among Department of Defense Beneficiaries by Race." *Cancer* 120, no. 19 (October 1, 2014): 3033–3039.

Fleming, Saroj, et al. "Black and White Women in Maryland Receive Different Treatment for Cervical Cancer." *PLOS One* 9, no. 8 (August 2014). https://www.ncbi.nlm.nih.gov/pmc/articles/PMC4133178/pdf/pone.0104344.pdf (accessed October 12, 2016).

Gale, Robert Peter, and Lax, Eric. *Radiation: What It Is, What You Need to Know.* New York: Vintage Books, 2013.

George, Prathama, et al. "Diagnosis and Surgical Delays in African American and White Women with Early-Stage Breast Cancer." *Journal of Women's Health* 24, no. 4 (2015): 209–217.

Goldner, Bryan, et al. "Incidence of Inflammatory Breast Cancer in Women, 1992–2009, United States." *Annals of Surgical Oncology* 21, no. 4 (April 2014): 1267–1270.

Grabler, Paula, et al. "Regular Screening Mammography before the Diagnosis of Breast Cancer Reduces Black: White Breast Cancer Differences and Modifies Negative Biological Prognostic Factors." *Breast Cancer Research Treatment* 135 (2012): 549–553.

Haji-Jama, Sundaes, et al. "Disparities among Minority Women with Breast Cancer Living in Impoverished Areas of California." *Cancer Control* 23, no. 2 (April 2016): 157–162.

Hamajima, N., et al. "Alcohol, Tobacco and Breast Cancer: Collaborative Reanalysis of Individual Data from 53 Epidemiological Studies, Including 58,515 Women without the Disease." *British Journal of Cancer* 87 (2002): 1234–1245.

Haslett, Michael J., et al. "Variation in Breast Cancer Care Quality in New York and California Based on Race/Ethnicity and Medicaid Enrollment." *Cancer* 122 (2016): 420–431.

Hershman, Dawn L., et al. "Household Net Worth, Social Disparities, and Hormonal Therapy Adherence among Women with Early-Stage Breast Cancer." *Journal of Clinical Oncology* 33 (2015): 1053–1059.

Hunt, Bijou R., Steve Whitman, and Marc S. Hulbert. "Increasing Black: White Disparities in Breast Cancer Mortality in the 50 Largest Cities in the United States." *Cancer Epidemiology* 38 (2014): 118–123.

Jacobs, Elizabeth, et al. "Perceived Discrimination Is Associated with Reduced Breast and Cervical Cancer Screening: The Study of Women's Health across the Nation (SWAN)." *Journal of Women's Health* 23, no. 1 (February 2014): 138–145.

Jolie, Angelina. "My Medical Choice." *New York Times.* May 14, 2013. http://www.nytimes.com/2013/05/14/opinion/my-medical-choice.html?_r=0 (accessed August 14, 2016).

Jones, Claire, et al. "A Systematic Review of Barriers to Early Presentation and Diagnosis with Breast Cancer among Black Women." *BMJ Open* (2014). http://bmjopen.bmj.com/content/4/2/e004076.abstract (accessed August 6, 2016).

Kimmick, Gretchen, et al. "Racial Differences in Patterns of Care among Medicaid-Enrolled Patients with Breast Cancer." *Journal of Oncology Practice* 2, no. 5 (September 2006): 205–213.

Kohler, Betsy A., et al. "Annual Report to the Nation on the Status of Cancer, 1975–2011, Featuring Incidence of Breast Cancer Subtypes by Race/Ethnicity, Poverty, and State." *Journal of the National Cancer Institute* 107, no. 6 (June 2015). doi:10.1093/jnci/djv048. https://www.ncbi.nlm.nih.gov/pmc/articles/PMC4603551/ (accessed October 1, 2016).

Knapton, Sarah. "Breast Cancer Breakthrough as Cambridge University Finds Gene behind Killer Disease." http://www.telegraph.co.uk/news/science/science-news/11336050/Breast-cancer-breakthrough-as-Cambridge-University-finds-gene-behind-killer-disease.html *United Kingdom Telegraph.* (accessed March 16, 2016).

Lehrer, S., S. Green, and K. E. Rosenzweig. "Affluence and Breast Cancer." *Breast Journal* 22, no. 5 (September 2016): 564–567.

Li, Lingyan, et al. "Emotional Suppression and Depressive Symptoms in Women Newly Diagnosed with Early Breast Cancer." *Women's Health* 15, no. 9 (2015). https://www.ncbi.nlm.nih.gov/pmc/articles/PMC4620014/ (accessed October 18, 2016).

Liu, Ying, Nhi Nguyen, and Graham A. Colditz. "Links between Alcohol Consumption and Breast Cancer: A Look at the Evidence." *Women's Health* 11, no. 1 (2015): 65–77.

Mayo Clinic. "Low Blood Cell Counts: Side Effect of Cancer Treatment." October 7, 2014. http://www.mayoclinic.org/diseases-conditions/cancer/in-depth/cancer-treatment/art-20046192 (accessed August 6, 2016).

McCarthy, Anne Marie. "Increasing Disparities in Breast Cancer Mortality from 1979 to 2010 for US Black Women Ages 20 to 49 Years." *American Journal of Public Health* 105, Suppl 3, (July 2015): S446–S448.

McDonald, Fiona. "The Science World Is Freaking Out over This 25-Year-Old's Answer to Antibiotic Resistance." *Science Alert.* September 26, 2016. http://www.sciencealert.com/the-science-world-s-freaking-out-over-this-25-year-old-s-solution-to-antibiotic-resistance (accessed September 30, 2016).

Miller, Kimberly D., et al. "Cancer Treatment and Survivorship Statistics, 2016." *CA Cancer Journal Clinics* 66 (2016): 271–289.

Mosavel, Maghboeba, et al. "Communication Strategies to Reduce Cancer Disparities: Insights from African-American Mother-Daughter Dyads." *Family Sys Health* 33, no. 4 (December 2015): 400–404.

Mukesh, Mukesh B., et al. "Randomized Controlled Trial of Intensity-Modulated Radiotherapy for Early Breast Cancer: 5-Year Results Confirm Superior Overall Cosmesis." *Journal of Clinical Oncology* 31 (2013): 4488–4495.

National Cancer Institute. *Chemotherapy and You.* Bethesda, MD: National Cancer Institute. 2011. https://www.cancer.gov/publications/patient-education/chemotherapy-and-you.pdf (accessed July 15, 2016).

National Cancer Institute. "Inflammatory Breast Cancer." January 6, 2016. Available online at http://www.cancer-gov/types/breast/ibc-fact-sheet (accessed May 4, 2016).

National Cancer Institute. "Managing Radiation Therapy Side Effects: What to Do about Mild Skin Changes." April 2010. https://www.cancer.gov/publications/patient-education/radiation-side-effect-skin.pdf (accessed August 5, 2016).

National Cancer Institute. *Surgery Choices for Women with DCIS or Breast Cancer.* Bethesda, MD. November 2012.

National Cancer Institute. *Understanding Breast Changes.* Bethesda, MD. February 2014.

National Cancer Institute. *What You Need to Know about Breast Cancer.* Bethesda, MD. April 2012. http://www.cancer.gov/publications/patient-education/wyntk-breast.pdf (accessed August 28, 2016).

National Center of Health Statistics. *Health, United States, 2015: With Special Feature on Racial and Ethnic Health Disparities.* Hyattsville, MD. 2016.

Nielsen, S. M., et al. "The Breast-Thyroid Cancer Link: A Systematic Review and Meta-Analysis." *Cancer Epidemiology, Biomarkers & Prevention* 25, no. 2 (February 2016): 231–238.

Norton, Amy. "Breast Cancer Health Center: Breast Cancer Survivors and Thyroid Cancer Risk." WebMD. 2015. http://www.webmd.com/breast-cancer/news/20150306/breast-cancer-survivors-may-have-higher-thyroid-cancer-risk (accessed October 10, 2016).

Oliver, M. Norman, et al. "Time Use in Clinical Encounters: Are African-American Patients Treated Differently?" *Journal of the National Medical Association* 93, no. 10 (2001): 380–385.

Pal, T., et al. "A High Frequency of BRCA Mutations in Young Black Women with Breast Cancer Residing in Florida." *Cancer* 121, no. 23 (December 2015): 4173–4180.

Palmer, Julie R., et al. "Predicted 25-Hydroxyvitamin D in Relation to Incidence of Breast Cancer in a Large Cohort of African American Women." *Breast Cancer Research* 18, no. 86 (2016). https://breast-cancer-research.biomedcentral.com/articles/10.1186/s13058–016–0745-x (accessed October 12, 2016).

Parise, Carol A., and Vincent Caggiano. "Breast Cancer Survival Defined by the ER/PR/HER2 Subtypes and a Surrogate Classification according to Tumor Grade and Immunohistochemical Biomarkers." *Journal of Cancer Epidemiology* (2014). https://www.hindawi.com/journals/jce/2014/469251/ (accessed April 22, 2016).

Parker-Pope, Tara. "Tackling a Racial Gap in Breast Cancer Survival." *New York Times.* December 20, 2013. Available online at http://www.nytimes.com/2013/12/20/health/tackling-a-racial-gap-in-breast-cancer-survival.html?pagewanted=all&_r=0 (accessed April 19, 2016).

Peek, Monica E., Judith V. Sayad, and Ronald Markwardt. "Fear, Fatalism and Breast Cancer Screening in Low-Income African-American Women: The Role of Clinicians and the Health Care System." *Journal of General Internal Medicine* 23, no. 11 (2008): 1847–1853. https://www.ncbi.nlm.nih.gov/pmc/articles/PMC2585682/ (accessed March 25, 2016).

Plasilova, Magdalena L., et al. "Features of Triple-Negative Breast Cancer: Analysis of 38,813 Cases from the National Cancer Database." *Medicine.* March 28–29, 2015, Presented at the Society of Surgical Oncology, Houston, TX. https://www.ncbi.nlm.nih.gov/pmc/articles/PMC5008562/pdf/medi-95-e4614.pdf (accessed September 16, 2016).

Rosenberg, Lynn, et al. "A Prospective Study of Smoking and Breast Cancer Risk among Africa-American Women." *Cancer Causes Control* 24 (2013): 2207–2215.

Ross, Jeffrey S., et al. "Comprehensive Genomic Profiling of Inflammatory Breast Cancer Cases Reveals a High Frequency of Clinically Relevant Genomic Alternations." *Breast Cancer Research Treat*, 154, no. 1 (November 2015): 155–162.

Rowland, Julia H., and Mary Jane Massie. "Breast Cancer." In *Psycho-Oncology*. 2nd ed., edited by Jimmie C. Holland et al., 177–186. New York: Oxford University Press, 2010.

Sheppard, Vanessa B., et al. "The Importance of Contextual Factors and Age in Association with Anxiety and Depression in Black Breast Cancer Patients." *Psychooncology* 23, no. 2 (2014): 143–150.

Shippee, T. P., et al. "Health Insurance Coverage and Racial Disparities in Breast Reconstruction after Mastectomy." *Women's Health Issues* 24, no. 3 (2014): e261–e269.

Sineshaw, H. M., et al. "Association of Race/Ethnicity, Socioeconomic Status, and Breast Cancer Subtypes in the National Cancer Data Base (2010–2011)." *Breast Cancer Research and Treatment* 145, no. 3 (2014): 753–763.

Sisti, Julia S., et al. "Reproductive Factors, Tumor Receptor Status and Contralateral Breast Cancer Risk: Results from the WECARE Study." *SpringerPlus* 4 (2015).

Siu, Albert L., on behalf of the U.S. Preventive Services Task Force. "Screening for Breast Cancer: U.S. Preventive Services Task Force Recommendation Statement." *Annals of Internal Medicine* 164, no. 4 (February 16, 2016): 279–296.

Smith, Grace L., et al. "Utilization and Outcomes of Breast Brachytherapy in Younger Women." *International Journal of Radiation Oncology* 93 (2015): 91–101.

Standish, Leanna J., et al. "Immune Deficits in Breast Cancer Patients after Radiotherapy." *Journal of Social Integrative Oncology* 6, no. 3 (2008): 110–121.

Stark, Azadeh, et al. "African Ancestry and Higher Prevalence of Triple-Negative Breast Cancer: Findings from an International Study." *Cancer* 116, no. 21 (November 1, 2010): 4926–4932.

Stead, Lesley A., et al. "Triple-Negative Breast Cancers Are Increased in Black Women Regardless of Age or Body Mass Index." *Breast Cancer Research*, 11, no. 2 (2009). http: breast-cancer-research.com/content/11/1/R18 (accessed May 10, 2016).

Stiel, Laura, et al. "A Review of Hair Product Use on Breast Cancer Risk in African American Women." *Cancer Medicine* 5, no. 3 (2016): 597–604.

Trivers, Katrina F., et al. "The Epidemiology of Triple-Negative Breast Cancer, Including Race." *Cancer Causes Control* 20, no. 7 (September 2009): 1071–1082.

Vachani, Carolyn. "Patient Guide to Tumor Markers." Penn Medicine OncoLink. April 28, 2016. http://www.oncolink.org/treatment/article.cfm?id=296& aid=560 (accessed May 6, 2016).

Wechter, Debra G. "Breast Self-Exam." MedlinePlus. February 27, 2016. https// medlineplus.gov/ency/article/001993.htm (accessed August 5, 2016).

Wolff, Antonio C., et al. "Recommendation for Human Epidermal Growth Factor Receptor 2 Testing in Breast Cancer: American Society of Clinical Oncology/College of American Pathologists Clinical Practice Update." *Journal of Clinical Oncology* 31, no. 31 (November 1, 2013): 3997–4013. http://jco.ascopubs.org/content/31/31/3997.full (accessed September 23, 2016).

Wright, Jean, et al. "Prospective Evaluation of Radiation-Induced Skin Toxicity in a Race/Ethnically Diverse Breast Cancer Population." *Cancer Medicine* 5, no. 3 (2016): 454–464.

Yilmaz, Sean, et al. "Use of Cryoablation beyond the Prostate." *Insights Imaging* 7, no. 2 (April 2016): 223–232.

Yoo, Jina H., et al. "Understanding Narrative Effects: The Role of Discrete Negative Emotions on Message Processing and Attitudes among Low-Income African American Women." *Health Communications* 29, no. 5 (2014): 494–504.

Index

Abdominoplasty, 39
Activities, 166
Ademywa, Foluso O., 4
Affordable Care Act, 19
Afinitor, 142
Africa, triple-negative breast cancer in, 57
African American Breast Cancer Alliance, 46
African American Women's Life Issues Today (Bradley), 71
Age: for breast cancer, 71; at diagnosis, 4
Agency for Healthcare Research and Quality (AHRQ), 79
Akinyemiju, Tomi, 98
Alcohol, 13, 14–16, 154, 156
American Cancer Society, 3, 6–7, 9, 13, 45, 46, 50, 58, 69–70, 73, 86, 87, 96, 100, 135, 146, 149; Cancer Action Network, 114
American College of Obstetricians and Gynecologists and mammogram age, 9
American Joint Committee on Cancer, 86
American Medical Association, 169
American Psychiatric Association, 15
American Society of Clinical Oncology, 58, 89
Andic, Fundagul, 54

Anesthesia, 81, 97, 101
Annals of Internal Medicine, 73
Antibiotics, 53
Anticonvulsants, 136
Antidepressants, 136, 137
Anti-estrogen therapy, 56, 58, 96, 137–42; adherence and income in black women, 140; aromatase inhibitors (AIs), 138–39; drug interactions, 137; hormone-blocking drugs, 138; vs. hormone replacement therapy (HRT), 138; side effects, 139
Anxiety, 31, 33–34; calming, 34; catastrophizing, 34; medication for, 34
Appetite loss, 134
Arimedex, 139, 141
Aromasin, 139
Aromatase inhibitors (AIs), 136, 138–39
Axxent, 119

Back or hip pain, 162
Belcade, 135
Betrayal by your own body, 31, 38
Biopsy, 23, 54, 58, 68, 73–74, 76, 79–83; before the biopsy, 80; core needle biopsy, 81–82; fine needle aspiration, 80–81; free-hand, 79–80; laboratory testing of, 80;

performance of, 80–82; questions to ask doctor, 83; results, 83; sentinel lymph node biopsy, 101; side effects, 82; stereotactic-guided, 79, 82; surgical biopsy, 81; time for result, 80; ultrasound-guided, 79
Black Women's Health Study, 16
Blame, 162, 164
Bleeding: from douching, intercourse, pelvic exams, 150; after menopause, 151; between periods, 150; vaginal, 162. *See also* Menstrual periods, long and heavy
Blood: cells, 123; clots, 134; coughing up, 149; in stools, 151; test tumor markers, 76–78
Blood test tumor markers: CA 15-3, 78; CA 27.29, 78; CA 125, 78; carcinoembryonic antigen (CEA), 76–77; tumor marker laboratory information, 78
Bone: damage, 136; density, 141; scan, 73, 75, 84; weakening, 139
Bowel: blockage, 151; emptying issues, 151
Bradley, Patricia K., 71
Breast: augmentation, 38; Cancer Genetic Study in African-Ancestry Population Initiative, 5, 57; Cancer Risk Assessment Tool, 59; and Cervical Cancer Prevention and Treatment Act, 19; exam, clinical, 67; implants, 24, 32, 109, 110–11; implants surgery, 110; lobes, 50; shape change, 162
Breast cancer: defined, 10; incidence in black women, by state, 51–52
Breast Cancer (American Cancer Society), 86
Breast cancer types, 49–63; basal breast cancer (*see* Breast cancer types, triple-negative); ductal carcinoma, 10, 50; ductal carcinoma in situ (DCIS), 50;

ER-negative PR-negative HER2/neu-negative breast cancer (*see* Breast cancer types, triple-negative); estrogen-receptor-positive, 16; hormone receptor positive, 10; inflammatory (IBC), 4, 49, 53–54; lobular carcinoma, 10, 50–51; lobular carcinoma in situ (LCIS), 50–51; triple-negative, 4, 10, 49, 54. *See also* Genetic classifications, triple-negative
Breast-conserving surgery. *See* Lumpectomy
Breastfeeding, 13, 32
Breast-sparing surgery. *See* Lumpectomy
Bruising, 53, 82

Caggiano, Vincent, 55, 56
California Cancer Registry, 55
Cancer, 112; *Causes Control,* 16; *Epidemiology,* 8, 98; *Medicine,* 16
Cancer, other forms, 146–59; cervical cancer, 149–51; checkups to identify, 147–48; colorectal cancer, 146, 151–52; death rate for black women, 146; lung cancer, 146, 148–49; origins in breast cancer, 147–48; thyroid cancer, 152–53
Cancer-related posttraumatic stress, 31, 37; medications, 37; symptoms, 37
Cardiopulmonary resuscitation (CPR), 169
Cataracts, 139
Centers for Disease Control and Prevention, 51, 68, 161
Cervical cancer, 149–51; and HPV, 149; Pap smear, 153; prevention, 149; rates among black women, 149; and smoking, 149; surgery rates in black women, 150; symptoms, 150–51; treatment, 151
Cervix, 149
Checkups, 160–61

Chemotherapy, 23, 24–25, 54, 56, 58, 96, 104, 116, 128–37; appetite, loss of, 134; bone damage, 136; cervical cancer, 151; colorectal cancer, 152; combinations of, 131; defined, 128–29; delays and race, 130–31; fatigue, 132; and fertility, 133; hair loss, 133; heart and cardiovascular damage, 134–35; lung cancer, 149; mental function, decreased, 134; nausea and vomiting, 132; neuropathy, 135; ovaries, damage to, 134; and pregnancy, 133, 134; questions for doctor, 136–37; side effects, 129, 131–36; timing of, 129–30; weight loss, 134

Chest pain, 149

Children, care for, 31, 35–36

Chills, 142

Cholesterol levels, increased, 139

Chowdhury, Rupak, 20

Clergy, 45

Clinical studies, 143–44; downside, 144; phases, 143

Colectomy, 152

College of American Pathologists, 58, 89

Colonoscopy, 147, 153–54

Colorectal cancer, 146, 151–52; rates among black women, 151; survival rate in black women, 151; symptoms, 151; treatment, 52, 152

Comments from people, dealing with, 46–48

Companion at doctor visits, 42

Compazine, 132

Congestive heart failure, 134

Control, 166

Contura, 119

Coughing, 148–49, 162

Coumadin, 80, 101

CT scan, 73, 75, 84

Cymbalta, 161

Cytoxic therapy. *See* Chemotherapy

Death: from cancer after surgery myth, 107; fear of, 107; rate, 8. *See also* Emotions, fear of death

Decadron, 132

Denial, 19, 21

Department of Defense (DOD) Military Healthcare System, 112

DeSantis, Carol E., 5

Diagnosis: of cancer, 3; questions to ask, 84; things not to do after, 11

Diagnostic and Statistical Manual of Mental Disorders (DSM-5), 15

Dialysis, kidney, 169

Diet, 25, 154, 155–56

Diphenhydramine, 137

Discharge: from nipple, 53, 69, 162; vaginal, increased, 151

Doctor, trust in, 34

"Do Not Resuscitate" (DNR) order, 168, 169

Drugs. *See* Treatment

Dryness, vaginal, 139

Education, 162–63

Effexor, 137

Elaxatin, 135

Embarrassment and breast cancer, 7

Emotions, 30–48; anger, 31, 33; anxiety, 30; anxiety and panic, 31, 33–34; betrayal by own body, 31, 38; black women, differences, 30–31; cancer-related posttraumatic stress, 31, 37; control, loss of, 31; depression, 30, 31, 36–37; emotional reactions, common, 31; expressing, 162, 163; fear, 30; fear for children, 31, 35–36; fear of death, 31, 32; fear of loss of feminity, 31, 32–33; fear of rejection, 31, 36; helplessness, 31, 37; sadness, 30, 36–37; shame and embarrassment, 31, 38–39

Endocrine therapy, 128. *See also* Anti-estrogen therapy

End-of-life issues, 168–70; continued treatment decisions, 168–69; decisions, 168, 170; "Do Not Resuscitate" (DNR) order, 168, 169; health care agent/medical surrogate/medical power of attorney, 168, 169–70; living will, 168, 169
Enewold, Lindsey, 112
Estradiol, 138
Estrogen, 10, 54, 55, 57, 58
Ethnicity and breast cancer, 4, 5–6
Ethnicity & Disease, 130–31
Etopoxide, 135
Examination, clinical, 67, 72
Exercise, 154, 157, 162

Family, telling, 44
Family history, 7, 11, 14, 89, 90, 107–8; and mammograms, 12
Fareston, 138
Faslodex, 138
Fatigue, 134, 149; from anemia, 151; chronic, 161
Fear, 30; for children, 31, 35–36; of death, 31, 32; of health care system, 19, 21–22, 39–40; of loss of feminity, 31, 32–33; of oncologist, 41–42; post-cancer, 162–63; of radiation from mammogram, 69; of rejection, 31, 36
Feelings, expressing, 162, 163. See also Emotions
Femara, 139
Feminity, 30, 32–33
Fertility, 133
Fever, 142
Florida Cancer Registry, 12
Food and Drug Administration (FDA), 143, 157
Friends and coworkers, telling, 44–45

Gale, Robert Peter, 69
Genetic analysis, 49

Genetic classifications, 54–55; BCL11A, 58; HER2 positive, 54, 56, 58–59; hormone receptors, 55; Luminal A, 54, 55–56; Luminal B, 54, 56; triple-negative, 54, 56–58
Genetic mutations, 12–13; BRCA1, 12, 17, 59–60, 74, 87, 89, 90; BRCA2, 12, 59–60, 75, 87, 89, 90; and MRI, 68
Genetic predisposition, 6
Genetics and black women, 5
Genetic testing, 7, 12, 89–90; and black women, 90; BRCA1, 12, 60; BRCA2, 12, 60; who should receive, 89
George, Prethibha, 103
Ghana, 57
Glucocorticoids, 136
Goldner, Bryan, 53
Grabler, Paula, 77
Grades of breast cancer, 89
Gynecologic checkups, 19, 147

Hair: loss, 125–26, 133; products, 15; thinning, 139
Halaven, 135
Headaches, 139
Health: care, lack of access to, 19–20; care agent/medical surrogate/ medical power of attorney, 168, 169–70; system, fear of, 19, 21–22, 39–40
Heart: arrhythmia, 134; problems, 139
Helplessness, 31, 37
Hemoglobin, 123
HER2. See Human epidermal growth factor 2 (HER2)
Herceptin, 55, 58–59, 141
Hershman, Dawn L., 140
Hip pain. See Back or hip pain
Hormone: receptors, 55, 57; replacement therapy (HRT), 138;

therapy rates among black women, 124

Hot flashes, 139

Human epidermal growth factor 2 (HER2), 54, 55, 58, 89, 90; and drugs, 141; testing, 58. *See also* Genetic classifications, HER2 positive

Human papillomavirus (HPV), 149; vaccine, 149

Hunt, Bijou R., 8

Hypertension, 134, 154, 156, 172

Ibrance, 142

Immortal Life of Henrietta Lacks, The (Skloot), 5

Infection, 82, 111

Insurance, 98, 109, 122

International Union against Cancer, 86

Internet, information from, 38

Ixempra, 135

James 5:14-16, 24

Jevtana, 135

Jews, Ashkenazi, 59, 89

Johns Hopkins Hospital, 5

Joint pain, 139

Jolie, Angelina, 60

Jones, Claire E., 23

Journal of: Clinical Oncology, 89, 90; *Oncology Practice,* 98

Kadcyla, 141

Kidney dialysis, 169

Kimmick, Gretchen, 98

Kuo, Jennifer Hong, 52

Kyprolis, 135

Lacks, Henrietta, 5

Lax, Eric, 69

Life expectancy, 146

Liu, Ying, 14

Living Beyond Breast Cancer, 46

Living will, 168, 169

Lobes of the breast, 50

Lump, 69, 152–53, 162

Lumpectomy, 60, 80, 95, 96–98, 99–100; appearance afterward, 100; breast feeling afterwards, 99; need for other therapies, 100; outpatient, 97; pain, 100; radiation, 114; and radiation, 118; rates in black women, 98; recovery period, 100; and recurrence, 97; scar, 97, 99; survival rate, 98

Lumps, 53

Lung cancer, 146, 148–49; non-small cell lung cancer, 148, 149; radiation, 149; rates among black women, 148; small cell lung cancer, 148; and smoking, 148; surgery, 149; symptoms, 148–49; targeted therapy, 149; treatments, 149

Lupron, 140–41

Luteinizing hormone-releasing (LHRH) analogs, 140–41

Lymph nodes, 84, 85, 87, 100; removal of, 108

Lymph vessels, 53

McCarthy, Anne Marie, 6, 89, 90

Male breast cancer, 76

Mammogram: abnormal, 76; age, 9; age and black women, 6–7, 12; diagnostic, 67, 68, 73, 74; digital, 67; dos and don'ts, 74; screening, 6–7, 23, 24, 25, 67, 72; screening and improved prognosis for black women, 77; screening guidelines, 73

MammoSite, 119

Marquibo, 135

Mastectomy, 38–39, 80, 95, 99–100; and abdominoplasty, 39; appearance afterward, 100; breast feeling afterwards, 99; and chemotherapy, 109; and lymph

nodes, 100–101; need for other therapies, 100; pain, 100; partial (*see* Lumpectomy); radiation, 109, 114; reconstruction surgery, 38–39; recovery period, 100; scar, 99; segmental (*see* Lumpectomy); sentinel lymph node biopsy, 101; sequence of events after, 109; simple (*see* Mastectomy, total); total, 100–101
Mastitis, 53
Medicaid, 130
Medical records, maintaining, 147
Meditation, 157
Menopause, 18, 139, 140
Menstrual periods, long and heavy, 151
Mental functioning, 134
Metastasis, 76, 85, 86
Moffitt Cancer Center, 12
Mood swings, 139
Mosavel, Maghboeba, 22
MRI of breast, 68, 73, 74–75
Myths about breast cancer surgery, 95–96, 106–9; death from cancer, 107; diet instead of surgery, 108; lymph nodes, 108; mastectomies and family history, 107–8; spread of cancer through surgery, 107; spread of cancer with knee or hip pain, 108–9

Nano-polymer, 143
Nasogastric tube, 168
National Breast and Cervical Cancer Early Detection Program, 19
National Breast Cancer Foundation, 50
National Cancer Institute, 51, 53, 59, 76, 83, 84, 98, 111, 119, 121, 122, 137, 142, 147, 149, 154, 155, 162, 165
National Institute of Alcohol Abuse and Alcoholism (NIAAA), 14
National Institutes of Health, 5
Nausea, 142; and vomiting, 122–23

Navelbine, 135
Neupogen, 123
Neuropathy, 135; chemotherapy-induced peripheral neuropathy (CIPN), 135
Neutrophils, 123
New Jersey Cancer Registry, 130
Nipple changes, 69. *See also* Discharge, from nipple
Nipples and reconstructive surgery, 110
Nolvadex, 137, 138
NSAIDS, 80

Obesity, 172
Oncologist: answers to your questions, 40–41; communicating with, 39; companion at visits, 42; fear of, 41–42; gynecologic oncologist, 151; handouts, ask for, 43; medical oncologist, 116, 151; notes from visit, 42–43; questions for, 40; radiation oncologist, 116, 151; summarizing, 41; surgical oncologist, 116; unsureness about your, 35
Oophorectomy, 139–41
Osteoporosis, 136, 139, 141
Ovarian: ablation, 139–41; cancer, 89, 90
Ovaries, damage to, 134

Pain, 69, 82, 100, 102–3; abdominal, 151; chronic, 161–62; and exercise, 162; joint, 139; post-cancer, 161–62; radiation, 122; during sex, 151
Painkillers, 102, 105
Pal, Tuya, 12
Panuplatin, 135
Papanicolaou, Georgios, 153
Pap smear, 149, 153
Parise, Carol A., 55, 56
Pathology, 24
Peek, Monica E., 21

Pelvic pan, 151
Perjeta, 141
PET scan, 75
Physical therapy, 106
Physician Data Query service, 83
Placebo, 144
Platinol, 135
Pomalyst, 135
Positivity, 162, 164
Post-cancer, 160–70; activities, 166; blame, 162, 164; checkups, 160–61; control, 166; education, 162–63; fatigue, 161; fears, 162–63; feelings, expressing, 162, 163; pain, 161–62; positivity, 162, 164; relaxation, 163–64; symptoms of concern, 162
Poverty, 19, 20–21, 171
Pre-cancerous conditions, 50
Pregnancies, 13, 17, 133, 134
Progesterone, 54, 55, 57, 58
Proton pump inhibitors, 136
Prozac, 137
Psycho-Oncology, 36

Quinaglute, 137
Quinidex, 137

Racism, 172
Radiation, 13, 16–17, 23, 54, 56, 96, 104, 114–27; before, 116–17; accelerated breast irradiation (APBI), 117, 126; appointments, keeping them, 115; and baldness, 125–26; blood cell counts, low, 123; brachytherapy, 118–20; breast changes and breast pain, 122; cervical cancer, 151; and chemotherapy, 116; colorectal cancer, 152; day of treatment, 119–20; effectiveness of, 126; explanation of, 115; external, 116; external beam radiation therapy (EBRT), 116, 117; fatigue or tiredness, 122; fear of in mammogram, 69; internal, 116; interstitial brachytherapy, 118–19; intracavity brachytherapy, 119; length of, 117; lumpectomy, 114; lumpectomy, after, 118; lung cancer, 149; and mastectomy, 114; myths about, 125–26; nausea and vomiting, 122–23; pain, 126; positioning, 117; questions for oncologist, 121; and radioactivity, 125; rates among black women, 114, 124; and recurrence rate, 118; side effects, 115, 120–24; and skin, 125; skin care, 119, 120–21; thyroid cancer, 153; timing for, 116; treatment, after, 119–24; treatments, other, 124; types, 116
Radiation: What It Is, What You Need to Know (Gale and Lax), 69
Rash, 162
Reconstructive surgery, 95, 96, 109–12; breast implant, 109; differences by race, 112; expenses, 111–12; and feeling in the breast, 109; implants, 110–11; and insurance, 109; and lumpectomy, 97; multiple surgeries, 110; nipples, 110; pros and cons, 110; tissue flap, 109, 111
Recurrence, 166–70; curable, 167–68; prolonging life, 168
Recurrence, prevention, 154–57; alcohol, 154, 156; diet, 154, 155–56; exercise, 154, 157; hypertension, 154, 156; smoking, 154, 156–57; spirituality, 154, 157; weight loss, 154–55
Recurrence rate, 56; and lumpectomy, 97
Relaxation, 163–64
Relaxation methods, 163–64; progressive muscle relaxation, 165–66

Religion, 24. *See also* Spirituality
Revlimid, 135
Risk factors for breast cancer, 11–18;
    access to health care, lack of,
    19–20; alcohol, 13, 14–16;
    behavioral, 18–19; breastfeeding,
    lack of, 13, 17; combined factors,
    19, 23; denial, 19, 21; ethnicity, 19,
    20; fear/mistrust of health system,
    19, 21–22; genetics, 13, 14, 18;
    gynecologic, 18; gynecologic
    checkups, 19; health care access,
    19; knowledge, lack of, 19, 22;
    medical issues, past, 18;
    menopause, 13, 18; menstruation
    age, 13, 17; obesity, 13–14; other,
    18; poverty, 19, 20–21;
    pregnancies, 13, 17; radiation, 13,
    16–17; smoking, 13, 16; spirituality,
    misguided, 19, 22; treatment
    factors, 18
Rosenberg, Lynn, 16
Ross, Jeffrey S., 54

Saline expander, 109
Savi, 119
Seattle Cancer Care Alliance, 59
Selective estrogen receptor modulators
    (SERMs), 138
Self-examination, 67, 69–72; and
    daughters, 71–72; how-to, 70–71
Serotonin reuptake inhibitors (SSRIs),
    137
Shame and embarrassment, 31,
    38–39
Sheppard, Vanessa B., 34
Shippee, T.P., 112
Shortness of breath, 148–49, 162
Sigmoidoscopy, 147
Sisters Network, 46
Skin care, 119, 120–21
Skin changes, 162
Skloot, Rebecca, 5

Smith, Grace L., 118
Smoking, 13, 16, 77, 148, 149, 154,
    156–57, 172
Spirituality, 19, 22, 154, 157, 172.
    See also Religion
Spouse or significant other, telling,
    43–44
Stages of breast cancer, 84–88; 0, 88;
    IA, 84, 88; IIA, 84, 88; IIIA, 84,
    88; IIIB, 84, 88; IIIC, 85, 88; IV,
    85, 88; importance of, 87; local,
    regional, or distant, 85; and
    survival rate, 87; TNM system of
    staging, 86–87
Stead, Lesley, 56
Stiel, Laura, 15
Stomach upset, 139
Stools, change in shape, 151
Support, emotional, 36
Support groups, 36, 45–46, 157, 172;
    survivors, 162, 163
Surgery, 23, 54, 56, 95–113; and
    additional therapies, 104; after,
    102–3; bilateral mastectomy, 23, 24;
    cervical cancer, 151; checkups
    afterwards, 113; colorectal cancer,
    152; day of, 101–2; delays and
    black women, 103; dos and don'ts
    before, 102; feelings about, sharing,
    106; lung cancer, 149; myths about,
    106–9; normal activities, return
    to, 104; pain, 102–3; painkillers for,
    102; pain medications, 105; and
    physical therapy, 106; psychological
    recovery from, 105–6; questions for
    yourself, 99; recovery from, 104–6;
    resting after, 105; second opinion,
    99; site, care of, 103; thyroid
    cancer, 153; types, 99–100
Survival rate, five-year, 4, 87,
    171–72
Symptoms of breast cancer, 67,
    68–69

Tamoxifen, 54
Targeted therapy, 128, 141–42; HER2, 141–42; hormone receptor-positive breast cancer, 142; lung cancer, 149; questions for doctor, 142; side effects, 142; thyroid cancer, 153
Taxol, 135
Taxotere, 135
Tests, preventive, 153–54; colonoscopy, 153–54; Pap smear, 153
Thromboembolic events, 134
Thyroid cancer, 23–24, 152–53; and breast cancer, 52; rates in black women, 52; symptoms, 152–53; treatment, 153
Thyroidectomy, 153
Tissue expanders, 110
Tissue flap, 109
Trastuzumab. *See* Herceptin
Treatment, 8–10; choosing, 39; drugs, 10; emerging, 10; inflammatory breast cancer, 54; and racism, 9. *See also* Chemotherapy; Radiation; Surgery
Tykerb, 141, 142

Ultrasound of breast, 67, 73, 74
U.S. Preventive Task Force, 9, 70, 73

Vaccines for breast cancer, 143
Valium, 132
Velban, 135
Ventilator, 169
Vitamin D, 167
Vitamins, 25

WebMD, 52
Weight: gain, 139; loss, 134, 149, 151, 154–55, 172
Wheezing, 149
Wigs, 133
Will, 170; living, 168, 169
Women's Health Issues, 112

X-rays and thyroid guard, 20

Yoga, 157, 165

Zofran, 132
Zoladex, 140–41

About the Author

Dr. Cheryl D. Holloway holds a PhD in public health. She is also a person who has experienced breast cancer twice and she is well aware of the issues black women face with cancer. Dr. Holloway is the program director for the Bachelor of Science in public health program at South University, a two-year program to assist students who wish to apply to the Bachelor of Nursing program and a four-year program for the Bachelor of Science in public health. The programs offer courses in microbiology, anatomy and physiology, human pathophysiology, chemistry, nutrition, and other preparatory courses. Supervising seven faculty members who teach science and public health, Dr. Holloway also teaches courses in health sciences, such as health promotion and wellness, issues in public health, and women's and minority health issues. Prior to Dr. Holloway's current position at South University, Novi, MI, she was an assistant undergraduate professor in healthcare management in Savannah, GA (2012–2013). She was also an adjunct graduate and undergraduate instructor at Central Michigan University (2006–2012).

Dr. Holloway wrote her doctoral dissertation on "Attitudes and Behaviors toward Early Breast Cancer Detection among African American Women in a Faith-Based Community," receiving her doctorate in public health in 2010. Dr. Holloway also holds a Master of Science from Central Michigan University in health administration in 2003 and a Bachelor of Science from Eastern Michigan University in sociology in 1994.

Dr. Holloway has been a volunteer for the American Cancer Society for more than 20 years, assisting women newly diagnosed with breast cancer.